Studies in Neuroscience, Consciousness and Spirituality

For further volumes:
http://www.springer.com/series/10195

Sangeetha Menon

Brain, Self and Consciousness

Explaining the Conspiracy of Experience

Springer

Sangeetha Menon
Consciousness Studies Programme
School of Humanities
National Institute of Advanced Studies,
Indian Institute of Science Campus
Bangalore
Karnataka
India

ISSN 2211-8918 ISSN 2211-8926 (electronic)
ISBN 978-81-322-1580-6 ISBN 978-81-322-1581-3 (eBook)
DOI 10.1007/978-81-322-1581-3
Springer New Delhi Heidelberg New York Dordrecht London

Library of Congress Control Number: 2013948741

Printed on acid-free paper

Springer is part of Springer Science+Business Media (www.springer.com)

Preface

Brain, Self, and Consciousness: Explaining the Conspiracy of Experience brings to its readers the view that to unravel what experience entails, is to place brain, self, and consciousness in an integral space. I take no shame or express less confidence in maintaining the absolute existence of the self. Perhaps it is my lifelong interest in, and commitment to, the Vedantic tradition that inspires me in this book to critically view the no-self, fleeting self and such nihilist and reductionist views about the self. While I am aware of the slippery ground of dualism that gets precipitated when the body-sense and self-sense are presented as discrete senses, I find such a distinction is inevitable to bring in the idea of the core-self that I propose in this book.

Brain, Self, and Consciousness argues that the central issue in brain studies is to explain the unity, continuity, and adherence of our experience, whether it is sensory or mental. To address such a unity is to understand the challenges that the brain and the self give each other. I use a cross-disciplinary framework guided by three disciplines, neuropsychiatry, philosophy, and psychology, to present my arguments. I hope this book will be a trailblazer in inviting philosophers, neurologists, and neuropsychiatrists to engage in a discussion on the duo of the brain and the self as the final frontier to understand the greatest and profoundest riddle of human existence, namely consciousness.

The primary reason for me to write this book was that only few books are available in the academic world that focus on a discussion on the concept of the self in the context of brain sciences and consciousness studies. And there are even fewer books that attempt a distinction between the body and self senses. I am hoping that this book will inspire scholars and students of philosophy, psychology and biology to extend the scope of the concepts of the body-sense and the self-sense and in the process develop the idea of the core-self.

The first notes that went into the shaping of this book were prepared during my visit as Shivdasani Fellow to the *Oxford Center for Hindu Studies* (Oxford University) in 2009. I am thankful to the air and space of Oxford and OCHS that exuded a charm and quietude that helped me start conceiving the ideas in this book. The time I spent in the picturesque environment of the *Indian Institute of Advanced Study* in Shimla as a Visiting Professor in 2013 helped me to go through the final manuscript with a fine-tooth comb. The availability of resources in plenty for reference is always a scholar's dream. I cannot thank enough the Library of the Institute where I work, the *National Institute of Advanced Studies* (NIAS), in Bangalore for making sure that I am always supported with easy access to a variety of reference material both online and print. Being in an institute like NIAS that favors interdisciplinary thinking and open questioning encouraged me to go beyond disciplinary confines in my thinking. If I was not a member of the NIAS family, perhaps this book would not have been possible!

The *Sambodh Center for Living Values* (SCLV) in Bangalore bestowed me with the idea of organicity of life through its mission and community work initiatives. By being a part of the Center I got to learn to be sensitive to life in much finer ways and discover untold joy every time a fruit tree bloomed or a bird nest was discovered. SCLV taught me that to discover the self is to listen to the subtle call of Mother Nature.

Finally, I record my heartfelt gratitude to my spiritual Guru and mentor Swami Bodhananda who introduced to me the concept of consciousness for my Research 25 years back. Without his vision on the centrality of the self and the ontological primacy of consciousness my study would have lacked an anchor. I am indebted to you, Gurudev, for helping me gain clarity in my thinking and humility in my beliefs. I dedicate *Brain, Self, and Consciousness* to you.

Contents

Biosketch of the Author

Sangeetha Menon is a Professor at the National Institute of Advanced Studies (NIAS), Bangalore, India, and heads the Consciousness Studies programme of NIAS. She is a nominated member of the International Society for Science and Religion (ISSR, Cambridge), a Board Member of the International Association for Transpersonal Psychology, and a Council Member of the Indian Council of Philosophical Research, Ministry of Human Resources Development, Government of India. Professor Menon has coedited the books, Consciousness, Experience and Ways of Knowing: Perspectives from Science, Philosophy and the Arts (2006); Science and Beyond: Cosmology, Consciousness and Technology in Indic Traditions (2004); Consciousness and Genetics (2002); and Scientific and Philosophical Studies on Consciousness (1999); authored Beyond Experience: Consciousness in the Gita, and coauthored Dialogues: Philosopher Meets Seer with Swami Bodhananda (2003). She has also co-edited a book "Nature & Culture" With Roddam Narasimha (2011). She has visited and spoken at many universities in India, the United States, England, Australia, Germany, France, Italy, Spain, Japan, Taiwan, Singapore, and Moscow. She was Visiting Fellow at the Oxford Centre for Hindu Studies, Oxford University, and at the Nanzan Institute of Religion and Culture, Nanzan University, Japan. She was invited to be a panellist at the World Parliament of Religions, Melbourne, in 2009. Apart from her academic interests, she writes poetry, fiction and is an avid photographer, artist, and web-designer. She also engages in charity programs, being a trustee of the Sambodh Foundation, India.

Chapter 1
The Problematic of Consciousness: An Introduction

> *This body is known as the object of knowledge, Arjuna; and the knower of the body is the self.*
>
> —Bhagavad Gita: 13.2

Biology and philosophy are the two disciplines that raise fundamental yet provoking questions about human life. The central question that these disciplines ask in the recent times is centred on the notion and experience of the self of the person. Today brain and the self are the two phenomena that everyone, from the common person to the scholar, is looking at to unravel the puzzle of consciousness. The belief is that somehow consciousness is connected with the self of the person. It is consciousness that presents to us experiences of joys and woes. It is also our dear self that is prone to the delicate functioning of the brain that directs the conscious states that you and I experience, and also the possibility of going into unconscious states due to neural dysfunctions. In all these the centre point is the experiencer along with the experience. It is the most intimate beholder of the experience that responds to the states of being conscious, and perhaps also to the states of unconsciousness.

While an important correlate of consciousness that all disciplines and all people are interested is awareness and different degrees of it, there are other aspects that connect consciousness and the self in finer ways. The character of the person, his or her ability to exercise choice, free will, and to take responsibility of acts and their consequences take us to the realm of wellbeing and how it is connected to the being of the person. Fundamental values that humans cherish such as truth, love and beauty are tied up with the deeper realms of our core-self, which are not amenable to reductionist filtering. Whatever theories of cognitive mechanisms we develop to explain the finer tastes and dispositions of humans, these very graces disappear when their causes and origins are explored. There is a cognitive closure that is confronted particularly when we discuss complex potentialities of the human self, such as eudaemonia, common good and altruism.

Because of the intertwined disciplinarity and complex psychological and spiritual possibilities involved, the question we ask—'what is consciousness?'—allures us without giving satisfactory definitions for all times. The 'what' of

S. Menon, *Brain, Self and Consciousness*, Studies in Neuroscience, Consciousness and Spirituality, DOI: 10.1007/978-81-322-1581-3_1,

consciousness is accompanied by 'where', 'when' and 'how' questions. Where is consciousness located, or what is the source of consciousness? When did consciousness emerge in the evolutionary stage of life? And, how is consciousness produced? The last question that is famously described as the 'hard problem'[1] (Chalmers 1995) leads to a 'harder problem'[2]of 'who is the experiencer' of the conscious experience. The 'who' of consciousness completes the circle by bringing in once again the 'what' of consciousness. We can respond to the 'who' of consciousness only in terms of definitions of consciousness. Is consciousness definable and knowable? As long as a 'knower' exists, can consciousness be completely, and in its entirety, known?

While the term 'consciousness' projects an immediate agnostic unknowability and mystery around it, gone are those days when discussions were limited to metaphysical and literary imaginations. The comeback of medicine and neuropsychiatry to understand the secret dispositions of the human mind and to travel the paths that the human self ventures in has helped begin a new revolution in the human sciences after psychoanalysis and Darwinian evolutionary theory. The new revolution is not about theorizing the strange and unacceptable behaviours of the child and the adult but presenting the varied possibilities of the person led by the neurochemistry of the brain and the willpower of the individual.

The coming together of neuroscience and neuropsychiatry has brought to light once again the biologically ridden body on one side and the delicate nature of the personhood on the other. Whether we question the exclusive focus given to neural structures and neural process to the exclusion of the rest of the anatomy in order to explain the mechanisms behind behaviours, attitudes and emotions, the progress in brain scanning technologies has made revealing patterns of how the human mind is intricately tied with the environment and the personality of the individual. What is strikingly interesting, if we span the discoveries and path-breaking studies in the last decade in neuroscience, neurochemistry and neuropsychiatry, is how the human personhood has resurfaced as an important factor that needs inclusion and explanation in a scientific manner. In the recent times it is with equal gusto that descriptions and presentations are made about cognitive processes, emotional valences and, most importantly, experience as an integral whole, in the alleys of science. Self is the puzzle for twenty-first century biology.

In the not-too-distant past, human experience and the subjectivity of the person were anathema for empirical sciences. Keywords that ruled a biologist's imagination were all inspired by the functional roles played by genetics and the physiology of the body. Only since two or three decades when qualitative attributes of experience and the personhood were brought into the laboratory to search for possible empirical

---

[1] David Chalmers divides the problem of consciousness into two: the easy problems and the hard problem. For discussion on this topic, see Sect. 3.2.1 in this volume.

[2] While the 'hard problem' is about 'conscious experience', I would suggest that the 'harder problem' is about the 'conscious experience'. For discussion on this topic, see Sect. 3.3.2 in this volume.

convertibles and biological correlates. In this trend which is now prevalent the first and foremost entrant was cognitive science. The cognitive sciences started with explaining the act of seeing in vision and such perceptual modalities that humans and animals possess. It was then found crucial to understand the intelligence behind the act of perception to justify the variations and differences in capabilities that individuals exhibit while interacting with the environment. Thus, 'mind' came into the forefront through the backdoor once again from the exclusive grips of philosophy and psychology. Along with the mind came in the new avatar of the body, which was seen as not completely biological but as partly conceptual and representational.

There are plenty of theories of embodiment available today in the discourse on mind and cognitive capabilities that have refashioned the understanding of the good old 'body' which classical biology was familiar with. The concept of the body in cognitive sciences is an extremely fascinating *subject* that has extended from the blood and flesh of the anatomical body to objects that we desire and possess, capabilities that we can 'afford', and most importantly to the self that inheres in the body. This means that the difference and distance between the traditional ideas about the body and the body-dweller are dwindling. The body is the subject and the living person. What is bereft of the body is given embodiment with powerful structures of phenomenology.

The impact of the body-phenomenology on sciences is such that emotions and psychological dispositions such as compassion have come to be regarded as significant in explaining the human self and its affective expressions. The affective sciences is today in par with the cognitive sciences to accommodate those tendencies of the human that was once considered to work against rational behaviour and appropriate decision-making procedures. The study of emotions and their place in the geography of the human self have also taken the alliance of the brain, its structures and neurochemical functions to present viable theories both within and outside the evolutionary context.

What does all this mean to that erstwhile philosophical gold mine of the 'self'? Is philosophy sidelined in the pursuit of the undisclosed engravings of the 'who' and the 'what' of the human self? Why have the body and embodiment become favourites of cognitive sciences to explain human capabilities? By bringing in the body from the dark corners of the pre-renaissance age to the modern show-light of cognitive sciences and information systems, have we pawned a few physical attributes of the body and added a few non-physical functions to it? Is the new avatar of the body taking away what is central to the existence of the self? In other words, is the 'body' of the recent times exhuming the self from the ancient times of metaphysics only to lead to its extinction?

These and many other subsidiary questions can be approached only if we bring into our focus the role of the interrelations between the brain and the self to chart the paths of consciousness and lead to the unknown and unimagined spaces of the possibilities of the human self. It is no more possible to have exclusivist presentations about the brain and the self if what we are looking for are the complex ways in which the human self is endowed.

Let us begin with one teaser for neuroscience – are *having a self* and *being a self* two different things? Many neuroscientists in the recent times have included 'self' as one of the questions science should answer to understand consciousness. But what is the scientific take on the self?

Often the self is conceived and conceptualized in the form of 'the self' or 'your self' or 'someone's self'. The form 'my self' is hard to be seen in cognitive sciences' repertoire. Once we accommodate the notion of self as 'my self', the detached and impersonal disregard for the self will reduce, and we will start talking about a living self that is you and me. This is the greatest difficulty faced by sciences such as neuropsychiatry. Since there is a lack of involved participation (of course, the practice of science cannot be involved to begin with!), even the most intimate subject of enquiry, the self, is overlooked, particularly its influence on every single person, even the person who is engaged in scientific enquiry. If at all such an intimate self is recognized, with no time spared, it is dismissed as a fleeting, promiscuous self that is the illegitimate child of sociolinguistics or information processing systems embedded in our brains.

The immediate availability of the bodily-self takes the centre stage of one's reflection to acquire closeness to one's identity. The body that inhabits the changing self becomes the self of the person. Let us examine this predicament further.

The physical body is governed by the principles of chemistry and biology. But when *I* and *my* body interact with the environment (the outside world of people, relations and objects) I do not worry or even think (unless one is a hypochondriac) how chemical processes are being executed in the body. What I think about are my feelings and thoughts that are directed from and to objects, people and relations. The physiological and anatomical processes of the body that are concealed from me, because of the human skin, are non-events for me. At the same time, somehow the brain and the body shroud the electrochemical processes with a unique biologically uncharacteristic feeling of *I and me*.

First, I am the one who thinks, feels and responds. Primarily it is the thinking person that relates to the body and is aware of the body. Subsequently, the feeling comes that *I have* a body. There is significant difference between the implications of a *being self* and a *having self*. The discussions on consciousness are yet to highlight this distinction that is basic to our experience. The experiential primacy of the self is closely tied up with our ability to reflect and introspect. While the brain might have a big say in deciding our states of waking, dreaming, conscious and unconscious states, it is the experiential self that has the capability to go deeper and reflect in a complex and focused manner.

The possibilities to discover the reified spaces of the self through reflection and meditative silence bring to us the concept of a core-self that is un-ideated and non-located. Since the focus is on sociocognitive interactions that humans (and other animals) are capable of, cognitive sciences and philosophy inspired by them endorse a fleeting self. But then the existence of the fleeting self itself is a product of the method that is used to arrive at its nature. Information systems–oriented methods, coupled with metaphysical nihilism, are best suited to caricature a self that is bereft of an ontological sustenance and used only for the purpose of justifying the meaningful nature of discrete events and the mind that is aware of them.

So, how do we approach the self and the body in ways in which there is more sophistication in our methods and better depth in our conceptualizations? The ways in which we fashion the idea of the self are certainly going to alter the ways in which consciousness presents itself to our minds.

This book raises a multitude of fundamental questions that connect human expressions (scientifically termed 'behaviour') with the body and the self. I engage in a critical appraisal to understand some of the mainstream thinking in neuroscience and neuropsychology on the ideas of the body, experience and consciousness. I hope to encourage open-ended thinking among readers to develop basic concepts for conceiving the exteriority of the self and interiority of the body, in the light of the studies on the subjective nature of consciousness. Some of the discussions I will engage in are:

- What is the body? Is it interior, exterior, or both?
- What is the self? Is it interior, exterior, or both?
- What are the body-sense and the self-sense?
- How is the body different from the self?
- Why is it important to distinguish the body from the self?
- Does experience belong to the body or the self?
- Of what is the body-sense constituted?
- Of what is the self-sense constituted?
- To which sense does 'experience' belong?
- What is experience? Who owns it? Who is the agent?
- Is there a minimal self?
- Is the minimal self sufficiently deep to retain the uniquely distinct human capabilities to reflect and introspect?
- Is there an extended self?
- Is the extended self a fiction that is created by narratives that are knitted according to our capabilities to imagine and confabulate?
- Is the self a 'bland' entity without any flavour or is it rich with feelings, emotions, perspectives, free will and purpose-orientation?
- What is the relation between being and wellbeing of the self? Are we mechanistic entities who have behaviours, controlled by genetically and environmentally determined factors?
- Who is a person? Are behaviourism and behaviour oriented approach adequate to represent the human self-hood? Is 'behaviour' an outdated expression with a biological overload and less humanistic tone?
- And most importantly, how does the brain challenge the self and the self challenge the brain?
- How is the conspiracy of 'experience' and the 'experiencer' created by the self-challenged-brain and the brain-challenged-self?

The nine chapters of this book are devoted to discussing one or more of these questions. All through the discussion, I underline the importance of considering brain-self interrelations, and also of separating the fleeting self of the cognitive and social sciences from the core-self that is deeply ontological. The discussion on the brain, self and the body is also expected to help separate mixed-up narratives inspired by phenomenology-induced embodiment and ontology-directed aspects of the core-self.

This chapter introduces the book to readers with a recount of the central issues and debates presented in the book.

Chapter 2 gives a preamble to the duo of the brain and the self. Self is the single unit of information and experience that connects sensations and emotions to consciousness. And the brain is the biological organ that is often treated as an agent and director of the body, guiding the working of sensations, emotions and consciousness. To be conscious is to be always associated with the neural apparatus. When on the one side human behaviours, attitudes and emotional capacities are intricately dependent on neural structures and mechanisms, while on the other these are guided by the experiential self. What is intriguing about the functioning of the brain is that neural connections are renewed and reconnected with newer experiences and as the environment demands. The brain seems to learn from its environment and at the same time is influenced by the initiatives that the self takes. There is a mutual challenge that is offered by the brain and the self. This challenge is to make possible the unity, continuity and adherence of our sensory and mental experiences.

The central puzzle that has fascinated researchers in consciousness studies is of the subjective nature of consciousness and how it emerges from brain structures and functions. The 'hard problem' of consciousness asks how discrete, quantitative, objective, neural processes that are spread out in the brain connect and combine to give rise to a unitary, qualitative, subjective, personal phenomenon close to all our lives. How does the quantitative input in terms of chemical and electrical signals give rise to a qualitative output whose nature is completely different?

Among the positions that try to solve the 'hard problem', one is that of the brain-mind identity. According to this position, consciousness and the self can be reduced to synaptic connections. Consciousness is all to do with the synaptic organizations in the brain. There is nothing other than the neural process. The neural process is the conscious experience. Consequently, the trend in line with this reductive explanation is the search for neural correlates of experiences and subjective dispositions. Technically called the 'neural correlate of consciousness',[3] or the 'NCC', approach, this line of search looks for causal connections between conscious experiences and neural correlates that are seemingly responsible for the origins of those experiences.

Functionalist theories, while questioning the need to frame consciousness for enabling an experience, make their arguments with the help of what is called 'unconscious perceptions'. For these theorists, consciousness is nothing other than sensations. All perceptions are unconscious, and sensations are a variety of actions. For instance, having the sensation of a red visual experience, moving the

[3] Neural correlates of consciousness are the minimal neural mechanisms jointly sufficient for producing a specific conscious percept. For further elucidation, see (Crick and Koch 1990).

hand, or calling someone, are actions of the same kind (Humphrey 2006). One of the criticisms against this view is that the brain does not have qualitative subjectivity and hence the brain and the perceptual experience cannot be identical.

Experience is the eye of the storm for the brain sciences and philosophies that study the self. In the Western world the significance of the body in conceptualizing and defining the self, inspired by Husserl and Merleau-Ponty (Merleau-Ponty 1964), was utilized in explaining consciousness by Francisco Varela (Varela et al. 1991). Embodiment theories are guided by the contention that the physicality of the body is insufficient to contain non-corporeal elements. We need to ask if the concept of the body and bodily experiences, even if extended beyond physicality, can contain the possibilities of non-intentional consciousness.

Two philosophical problems that arise from the analysis of experience are the inherent subject-object divide, and the degree of the 'other' in 'me' and that of 'me' in the 'other'. We might possess an intuitive sense of the other, but it is not easy to have a well-articulated description of oneself. The slippery problem that underlies the first-person nature of consciousness is the entanglement of the body-sense and the self-sense in it, which also forces us to revisit the subject-object divide time and again. It is important to examine both these senses. Are the body-sense and the self-sense distinct, and if so what demarcates the distinction? Where and how are these senses entangled? What constitutes the basic everyday senses that we possess in a default mode?

In Chap. 2, I also discuss the puzzles surrounding consciousness that will stay for another decade or more. The ongoing discussions that address the 'unity' of consciousness, especially in the field of cognitive sciences, suggest two concepts as significant in understanding the binding nature of consciousness. These are 'intention' and 'agency'. Our consciousness is intentional when we desire and when we act. We are the agents of our acts. Brain and the self together knit the framework of intention and agency to make events and experiences possible. Such a framework has helped the shift of scientific focus from 'a biological organ for consciousness' to 'a situated brain'.[4]

How does consciousness emerge from the complex biochemical molecules and electrical impulses in the brain? Or is consciousness an emergent product at all? In Chap. 3, I present a brief profile of consciousness with both biological and philosophical accounts. The reason for the brain to be rated as the most important organ of the body is its incredible complexity, unpredictability and malleability. Neuroscience started in the eighteenth century as phrenological studies, the only known scientific way to understand the brain, and it has today progressed with advancements in brain scanning equipment and brain mapping. The brain is

[4] Traditionally, life sciences recognize 'consciousness' not as a qualitative entity but as a function of brain and its processes. Hence, consciousness is a biological entity. For the past two or three decades, the rising number of works in neuropsychology and cognitive sciences encourage a shift in this perspective. Consciousness and brain cannot be viewed merely as physical and biological entities. The brain is guided by the cognitive and mental processes and therefore is situated within a culture and within the individual's life experiences.

mapped by various ways to charter the content and cause of experiences ranging from deception to compassion. A score of allied disciplines have emerged, such as neuropsychiatry, neuropharmacology, neurotheology, all centred on the physiology of the brain but extending conceptually from biological to philosophical and psychological concepts and correlates.

While charting various pathways, these disciplines overtly ask the questions 'who is the owner of consciousness?', and 'what are the implications for the self?'. While now and then theories about the nature and origins of the experiencing self are floated, most of them are debunked because of the lack in philosophical depth. While it is beneficial for the neurosciences to endorse a fleeting self fictitiously produced somewhere in the warps of the neural networks, such a conception cannot explain forces of deeper humanistic concern such as wellbeing. It is not easy to dismiss the possibility of a lasting self that is responsible for invoking phenomena such as self-healing and self-transformation.

The philosophical discussion which has ensued in the circles of post-Cartesian mind-body dualism has embraced a different sort of idealism and empiricism that either dismisses the possibility of a core-self, or equates neural functions with subjective qualities. Thus, there is either only a fleeting self, or the brain itself is the experiencer and agent. The Cartesian distinction of the mind from the body was an offshoot of the scientific revolution of the seventeenth century and it was important to highlight the mind as an independent source of knowledge, and the body as a conscious automaton. Twenty-first century philosophy-neuroscience nexus has almost given up this schism but has embraced a reductionist model that is either biologically laden or philosophically extreme. Many attributes of the classical concept of the mind are now transferred to the body and the brain. Embodiment theories help to extend the idea of corporeality and exteriority, but also fall prey to an extreme physicalization of non-physical entities. And the first in this row is the self. The existence of the self is often identified with the possibility of it embodying another object or an action. Or, the self is identified with the body itself. Thus, what we have today is a different kind of debate which is far from the simple dualism inaugurated by Descartes in the West. This debate can be described as the 'body-mind and body-self' debate.

The 'hard problem', which brought to light the unease in suggesting a biological escape for subjective consciousness, bargains for a unitary self. Now, there is a divide between what can be achieved through understanding the physiology and perceptual mechanisms of the brain, and finding out how the discrete neural processes are bound together to give rise to a neatly unified sense of 'my experience'. Perhaps such a divide is beneficial for reaching conceptual clarity, and gaining humility, on what the empirical methods of science can attain. The conceptual clarity that is unavoidable for any study on consciousness is the distinction between 'being conscious' and 'what is responsible for consciousness'. The first is experiential and is marked by the overflow of subjective qualities. The second is empirical and sophisticated tools have been designed to find out how consciousness emerges, or, the causal mechanism behind the subjective experience. For sure, we can know how experience and knowledge happen with the help of neural pathways charted and biochemical molecules isolated. But to reduce the knower into the known and then to say the knower also is biologically produced involves a simplistic but grave categorical mistake. The knower can never become the known. The existence of the knower is imperative for something to be known.

Recent research in neurogenesis has suggested that the brain is prone to change at all times, and that synaptic activity is modified by new learning. The brain has the ability to transfer, extend and take over functions. The astonishing revelation of the recent times is that the brain remodels throughout one's lifetime. The capability of the brain to structurally and functionally reorganize according to demands of changes in the environment adds to the philosophical puzzle surrounding consciousness and self-identity. Chapter 4 explores the philosophical riddles and experiential ironies that are presented to us by the non-rigid brain. Along with the enigma of the fluid nature of the brain is another equally difficult phenomenon to understand. This is: how does the self make sense of the neural changes and create corresponding changes in sensations and personal identity? Just as there are neural correlates of consciousness which are biologically derived, are there correlates of the self that are capable of altering the neural pathways in curious ways? Can we identify positive thinking, self-effort, love, compassion and spiritual quietude as the correlates of a deeply placed self? Emerging interest in the area of 'contemplative sciences' points towards the advantageous impact of reflection, meditation and positive imagining on one's wellbeing.

One of the foundational pillars in cognitive sciences, particularly in theories of social cognition, is what is technically called 'theory of mind'. 'Theory of mind' is the capability we all possess in varying degrees of imagining and knowing what the other person knows. Our social encounters in daily life work in meaningful, predictive and purposive ways because we operate with the help of the 'theory of mind', which gives crucial information about the minds of the people we meet and interact with. It is also because of the 'theory of mind' that we are able to distinguish between private mental states and information that is shared or commonly available.

What I propose in this chapter, in order to build on the 'theory of mind', is the fundamental divide between the 'me' and the 'other' that we carry with us in our social living. The 'me' and the 'other' are cognitive structures on which are embedded all human acts, desires and intentions. What is 'the me and the other' divide? I have a sense that is physically supported and mentally guided as 'me' which gives me an immediate recognition of the limits of my personal-identity. The 'me' sense is invariably accompanied by what is other-than-me based on my preferences for inclusion and exclusion of people, objects and life around. Since it is not solely directed by the limits of the physical body but is very much influenced by the capability of individual consciousness to include and accept, different people have different degrees of this divide. As we age and move ahead in life, we cultivate newer values, world views, and perspectives about our own selves. With these crucial additions and modifications, our me-and-the-other divide also changes, leading to either a narrowing down or widening of the divide. We either include more in our 'me' or in our 'other'. As we include more in our 'me' the divide becomes narrower. The narrowing of the divide has both detrimental and beneficial effects. The beneficial effect is the ability to see the unity in the universe and embrace a universal brotherhood. The danger is what is identified in psychopathology as delusion and absence of self-reference and self-identification. It is important for us to know the extremities of our 'me' and 'the other' so that there is no collision in psychological and physical interactions. Dysfunctions of the brain and the mind can dangerously alter the me-and-the-other divide, causing havoc to self-perception.

While the 'theory of mind' and the me-and-the-other divide help us to model another self, in order to understand and be sensitive to one's own self what is needed are awareness and the ability to introspect and reflect. There are theories about grading perception of one's identity using degrees of awareness and self-recognition. The ability to self-reflect helps the person recognize oneself in a grounded and inclusive manner. The prevalent misperception that occurs in biology-inspired theories of self-recognition is that reflection is a modification of the ability to recognize oneself (in the mirror). Self-recognition is mostly a perceptual ability combined with a self-identification process. The ability to reflect comes from a different school and needs the invocation from the core-self. The core-self guides two functions of consciousness. There is an outward movement as well as inward movement of consciousness. This is the reason that some of the Eastern schools of philosophy like the Vedantic tradition maintain the possibility of non-intentional consciousness.

Some biologically inspired questions that paved the way for the discovery of 'mirror neurons' were: 'Are there common processes and ingredients in the "me" and the "other"'? Will that which happens in the 'other' influence my 'me'? At the least neural theories about mirror neurons tend to argue that there are shared neural centres in us that get activated while we perform and act while we see another individual performing the same act. The psychological phenomenon that corresponds with the function of mirror neurons is what is called 'empathy'. Empathy is the ability to get into the shoes of the other and feel what the other feels and experiences. We can immediately see that the 'theory of mind', the me-and-the-other divide, self-reflection, and empathy all are phenomena that spring from the master intelligence of the joint work of the self and the brain.

Yet another important component of our psychological repertoire which is influenced by the functions of the brain is the system of memory. Our ability to connect the past to the present and the future is because of the short stories that we store in our minds about people, objects and relations that come into our interactive space. Memories are engrained in such complex and intricate manner that at times perception, touch or smell brings in a barrage of experiential content to us from the past. The exciting philosophical debate on memory is about determining the 'truth' behind memory. How much of memory is true to the corresponding original experience? And how much of the 'me' to whom the original experience incur is stored in the memory? How much meaning is shared between the original experience and the recalled memory about it? Is the system of memory-making a step towards the effort of the brain and the self for meaning-making? Without memories and their recall do our experiences count as meaningful as they are?

How are sensations presented to our awareness? The mechanism of the memory system tells us that we do not have raw sensation. Sensations that we experience are coloured by the associations we have made in the past. Experiences are the aftermath of a filtering process through feelings, attitudes, beliefs, value systems, memories and the self-narrative. Self-awareness, coupled with the information received from 'the other' through the models we simulate and representations we form, function as the subjective marker that makes meaning out of an event or an act. The not-so-rigid brain gets feedback when our 'me' sense and 'the other' sense coexist and pervade into each other without losing the defining characteristics of each world.

But, what is the 'me' sense? Is it a sense that sprouts from the body or the self? Chap. 5 analyses the concept of 'sense' itself and the constituents of the body-sense and the self-sense. The question that I ask is: 'Is my inner awareness of my-self separate from my body'? While there are imaginative views about the different existences of the self such as embodied, minimal, autobiographic, synaptic, fleeting, thin, there is hardly any detailed account of the experiential self, the self that we possess and carry with us—or, perhaps, the self that carries us!

The mainstream view about the self is that it is a grand representation that the mind and brain together create, and hence the sense of the self is a special kind of feeling. On finer analysis, we find that the 'feeling' and representation that is conceptualized relies mostly on the attributes of the body and its corporeality that mark all experiences. For this reason, I endeavour to provide a distinction between the body-sense and self-sense in this chapter with the argument that the self-sense cannot be grouped under the category of precepts and sensory feels. In order to understand the nature of our identity with body parts, and body as a whole; to recognize the illusoriness and reality of that (phantom) body part which we own as ours, to relate to the representation of the body and its changing contours, we need to distinguish between the body-sense, the self-sense and also imagine the possibility of a core-self which is inclusive and beyond the binary.

The body-sense that is given to us in an almost default mode is a combination of internal and external sense functions such as pain, balance, thirst, hunger, vision, taste, touch, smell and hearing. Through the panoply of these senses and the mental structures we relate with the external and internal world. At the same time, our natural capabilities to gauge pressure, weight and space as required when our bodies come in touch with other objects (proprioception) and the ability to demarcate the space needed around our bodies (peripersonal space) bring the body to bear our action, movement and interactions in a social world. Our body has the capacity to intuitively 'know' how much space it requires, for instance to occupy a seat, to maintain a distance that is not too distant and not too near from the person with whom we interact. How does the body 'know' and operate these physiocultural mechanisms seamlessly? A strong theory that responds to this question holds the view that the brain creates topographic maps that are continuously updated with the help of feedback from personal habits and day-to-day encounters. With the help of the body maps the brain too gives 'feedforward' to the body to perform in an optimal manner. In effect, our experiences change the maps in the brain, and with reorganized body maps in the brain our experiences also get altered. What is even interesting is that the brain maps not only the physical body, but also the space around the body, which houses objects, tools we use, people with whom we interact and many other socio-cultural expressions. The peripersonal space, which is a subject of neurological interest of recent origins, extends our physical body-sense to embody people, objects and other entities and make a connection to feel and identify with these. How subjectivity is inhered in the body-sense to a great extent perhaps can be unravelled if we build upon the possibilities of the peripersonal space.

The next level of what constitutes the body-sense extends the idea of physicality to cognitive structures of action-initiation and action-identification. Which means, we are the agents of our actions, and we own our actions. Agency and ownership are features of the body-sense which makes the latter compatible for engaging in action and relating subjectively to its outcomes. Studies in neuropsychiatry tell us that brain lesions and brain dysfunctions can cause major impairment to the sense of agency and owning actions and body parts. While schizophrenic patients often report delusory events for which they do not take authorship and ownership, patients of asomatognosia disown or neglect body parts. The balance between the body-sense and the body-absence is delicately marked by the way in which the neural maps and functions are organized in normal conditions and conditions that ensue from brain and psychiatric dysfunctions.

Any experience is given in an intact manner for the experiencer because of the self-sense. It is because of the self-sense that one is able to move from one experience to another and collate different experiences. It is this sense which helps us recognize the same person who was in the past moment, who continues to be in the present and might be there in the future. We cannot say that the self-sense is a sort of memory or a representation because it is that sense which has to be beyond all the other structures of mind in order to illumine as belonging to one integral whole of the person. With the self-sense we become agents of action, possess intentions, make choices and are responsible for the choices we make. Self-sense is an indivisible, continuous and organic intuitive sense that accompanies our lives without fail.

Recent discussions on the self focus on the fleeting and functionally minimal self. Can we derive a self that is minimal and which can be identified in a machine or in an animal? The minimal self query looks for the very basic, stripped down self. While this project is worthwhile to understand the primary ingredients of the self, it also creates the impression that the sense of the self is a phenomenon that can be cut into parts of increasing order. If we hold that the self-sense at any time is organic, then to talk about the minimal self will have no meaning. Another prevalent notion is the narrativistic idea about the self. Self-sense is a story that is continuously made and told to oneself, according to this view. Such a self is dependent on language and on our ability to tell stories. One of the most provocative concepts of the self in the recent times has been that of the 'ego tunnel'

(Metzinger 2009), which completely negates the self saying that it is a myth and therefore non-existent. To argue for the non-existent and shifting sense of the self, several variations of intersensory, illusion-based studies are used.

To equate the self-sense as an emergent of the feedback received by the brain from vision, vestibular, tactile and proprioceptive capabilities is to limit oneself to just a being who sees and uses the body for sensing location and locomotion. In Chap. 5 I further explore why the minimalism project is an insufficient method in fabricating a primitive self if what we are interested is the self-sense that comes as an integral whole, which is alive and organic at any point of time. I propose the core-self as a response to the entanglement of the body-sense and the self-sense.

With a proposal for the core-self, in Chap. 6 I trace the contours of the self in the context of challenges caused to the self-sense in neuropsychiatric disorders, and how seeking of meaning and purpose becomes important. Our experiences tell us that the boundaries of self-sense are flexible, contributing to better or worse existences. The self at times can be fractured or become fragile. The psychiatrically and neurologically challenged self finds it difficult to sustain oneself and the encounters in a socio-cultural world. The self for some others is the most encompassive and inclusive phenomenon leading to self-actualization. The spiritual self is that which includes everything.

In the cases of neuropsychiatric challenges that cause strange self-ascriptions, what strikes us is the self's capacity to make meaning of what is experienced, even when the brain circuitry is severely damaged. It is because of the core-self that the individual constantly tries to solve dilemmas even when they are neurally created. This also implies that the more the core-self is invoked the better the chances for self-recovery.

In spite of the oddities and differences in and through experiences, an overall value of the self-sense stays that carries forward the agenda of seeking purpose, thereby achieving meaning. It is undeniable that there is a continuity in all our experiences which brings forth the past, present and future to the same moment. We think using information from the past and expectations about the future. The memories that we form are closely connected and contiguous to our experiences. It is the continuity that is felt as adhering to a single unit of consciousness which we call as my-self. Contrary to the Cartesian dictum 'I think, therefore I am', in our daily life we first *are*, and therefore are able to do many things, mental and physical. Otherwise all our physical and mental acts will not have a place to adhere to and will be floating around. The question that arises from the central place that self has in our experiences is: Are our abilities to find meaning and unify and integrate different experiences a function of the brain or the self? What I postulate is that it is the core-self, the deeper and complex realm of our being, which is impervious to our methods of knowledge, that helps generate meaning.

The body image and the limits of the body-sense are susceptible for modifications based on alteration in social perceptions, brain structures and functions. Even while experiencing the shifting contours of the body and self-senses, that entity which perceives, intents and makes decisions, however weird they are, is primary and is the pre-experiential, pre-conceptual core of the self-sense. Where we fail in theorizing the self is when we hold the faulty assumption that the body-image itself is the self-sense and creates ownership of the body. The concept of ownership that we discuss in the context of the body is primarily engaged to theorize discrete acts that are directed by proprioceptive abilities. The 'feeling' that my body is owned by me is itself a deeper sense that ensues from the core-self. It is because of a deeper being of the core-self that the altered body maps get translated into meaningful or strange experiences, all of them owned by a singular I-am-ness. For this reason it is essential to distinguish between the self-sense and the body-sense and both from the core-self. The uniqueness of one's perceptions and experiences are not the result of these being connected to one's body but because of the underlying core-self. My key argument in this chapter is that the core-self is the very core of being from where everything else, the body and the other, 'me and the other', seem to rise, reside and disappear. However much we attempt to subjectivize the body and the body-sense, these cannot become the core-self.

Chapter 7 discusses emotions as the affective markers of experience. Emotions carve our personal identities. Without emotions in us, others will find it hard to understand us and communicate with us. The bridge for social interactions is built by emotions which play the role of narrators of physical, mental, and social health for oneself and for others. When from one point of view emotions guide neural mechanisms for physiological and chemical balance, from another viewpoint emotion enhances self-expression and the presentation of the person.

Emotion has been a subject of serious interest in public lives and intellectual curiosity since the time of Egyptian and Ayurvedic medicine. The study of emotion brings in the role of the brain, the body, and the self, interspersed by the influence of environment, society, art, and one's character. Why and for what outcome does the brain generate emotions? Should we consider emotions as evolutionary vestiges or as those subjective elements of personal significance that enhance experience? How are feelings and emotions different? Are feelings always dependent on sensations? Are there feelings that are not dependent on sensations? Can feelings be considered as discrete cognitive events and understood within the framework of neuroscience? Another pertinent issue that is discussed currently is the ability of emotions to be part of a decision-making process by contributing to the cognitive deciders. Such a conception of emotions is important for our analysis if we are only cognitive entities, and if we think exclusively as rational entities. Do emotions influence our cognitive capacities and rational processes?

Physical sensations and mental feelings are presented in a united manner to the subjective experience. There is a belongingness and a sense of owning about feelings. One of the ways in which emotions are theorized is with the help of the concepts of qualia and representationalism. What makes an experience unique to the person is defined by its qualia and therefore mostly inaccessible to others. The closest relative to qualia is emotion because of its person-centric nature. For many neuroscientists the concept of emotion is one of the junctions where brain and personal experience meet. Emotions are pervasive phenomena interconnected with physiological mechanisms and phenomenal meanings in experiences, and give us the feel factor through anatomical features (such as 'gut' feelings) and psychological aspects. As unique individuals, we own and express different degrees of emotion, and thus some of us are described as 'warm' persons and some others as 'cold'. Often the degree of experience and expression of emotions is decided by the repertoire of our capabilities, dispositions such as our beliefs, desires, attention, and sensitivity to nuanced meanings, conceptualization and visualization.

A greater challenge in theories about representation of emotions is the inadequate inclusion of the role of bodily subjectivity in framing the continuum of self-experience. Philosophers who hold a strong representationalist view defines the phenomenal character of an experience as one and the same as its poised, abstract, non-conceptual, intentional content. The content of qualia is non-conceptual and is not neurophysiological, according to the emergent theory. Along with the representation theories there are also contesting views that emotions do not have definable boundaries in the brain or the body. We can only presume that the feel is a property of subjective experiences which is invoked by the object. While the feel factor is dependent on the object and the personality of its beholder, feel also has universal accompanying features such as ownership and an assuring sense of being related to the experienced world. Without feeling emotions and expressing them we cannot communicate with ourselves let alone with others. The delicate nature of emotions aside, without feelings we cannot accurately assess the inner worlds of others and ourselves, cannot bring in creative and imaginative outpourings and enrich our personalities. The feel factor of emotion is the unavoidable face of consciousness whichever way it is conceived theoretically, as basic, or pluralistically nuanced.

Our natural ability to express a variety of feelings and at the same time conceptualize our feelings cognitively into the rational structures of thinking indicates that the self that we possess and cherish is somehow influenced by beliefs, hopes, attitudes, values, etc. We seek our wellbeing through acts of choice and the exercise of free will. In Chap. 8, I discuss the relation between the being and wellbeing of the self, and how it is important to invoke the core-self to gain meaning and purpose in living.

Several mainstream positions in neuroscience support a self that has no abiding existence. The central challenge that the 'fleeting self' or 'no self' theorists have to address is how we account for the character and moral agency of the person. Character cannot be imagined to belong to a person with no self or fleeting self. Hence, do moral agency and free will have to be understood as special kinds of virtue that cannot be explained adequately with the help of a culture of fleeting behaviours and changing perceptions of the person?

The possibility of character to belong to only a self that has been continuous, and which feels responsible not only for the initiation of acts but also for the outcomes cannot be ruled out. It is hard to understand how a person with fleeting or no self can be held responsible for intentions, acts and consequences. Our sense of freedom to make choices without being biased by favourable or unfavourable outcomes indicates that the human mind is not a blank slate, and that the self is not a product of language and changing environment. Character and the self are to be seen in a common space of existence if we have to appreciate that human consciousness possesses deeper levels of reflective capability and the ability to relate to an undefined core-self at times of challenges to the physical and mental aspects of one's identity. We admit that behaviours are expressions of one's character nourished by the virtues that are treasured.

There is a renewed contemporary interest in old values such as empathy and compassion, though there is an equal effort to trace their biological foundations in mirror neurons and brain-maps. Such a trend invites us to think about the phasing out of stark divisions between 'me' and the 'other', and to include more of the 'other' in 'me'. Cultural neuroscience, social emotions, place of emotions in decision-making, and most importantly details about the self-sense, its peripheries and the ontic core gain serious attention, raising questions such as: How much of the self-sense is embodied? Is the self-sense separable from body-schema and its proprioceptive capabilities? What is the role of ownership and agency in binding the self-sense to the body-sense? What is the nature of the self-sense in people with acute impairments in movement and touch senses? Is the self-sense primarily a meaning-making mechanism that overrides bodily limits and disabilities?

Values and virtues are the signposts that confirm the existence and workings of the self. To study self is to study the self-sense, its dysfunctions and causes, its ability to cope with psychosomatic challenges, feedback mechanisms between the self-sense and the body-sense, and one's search for new meanings. The subjective self through his or her experiences, values, attitudes and self-perceptions can alter or influence neural changes to bring in qualitative progress in life. There is little doubt that the brain and the self are the final frontiers of consciousness.

The individual unique stories of our selves are designed by the values and beliefs we cherish, attitudes and perceptions we covertly possess, and memories that run through our thoughts, influencing our judgements. A complex set of personal and interpersonal entities are harboured in our selves, in the course of a day, due to which we feel secure at times, insecure at other times. We constantly search for our notion of wellbeing. We believe that through the course of the day's activities we will be led to a being-well state. So, are we seeking pleasure? The primary distinction between pleasure and happiness (wellbeing) is that the existence of pleasure borrows significant content from sensations, whereas happiness is a deeper feeling that is invoked from the undefined core-self. Pleasure is dependent on objects, people and situations. Wellbeing is dependent on the inner disposition of the individual, his or her sense of autonomy, virtues and passion for common good. Wellbeing mostly is experienced in our lives when we find a meaning and purpose to living. In almost all of wellbeing studies the two life traits that clearly emerge are 'meaning' and 'purpose'. I discuss in this chapter some of the ideas on the origin of meaning, primarily whether it is person-centred or society-centred.

In Chap. 9, I explore the final frontiers in understanding consciousness, and pose the question whether we can move beyond the brain and the body. The central puzzle that consciousness studies presents to us is the existence of the evading agent and the enjoyer in and behind the experience. How does the subjective intimacy of the self and experience gets created by an organ that is directed by neurochemical mechanisms? Neuroscience employs brain imaging techniques, encephalographs, radioactive tracer dyes, clinical diagnostic tests, cognitive and artificial intelligence experiments to trace the beginning and end of the agent of action and the enjoyer of experience, knowing fully well the possibilities and limits of these methodologies.

The central concern of this book is to enquire how the brain and the self conceive their role-play and create the conspiracy of experience, where the physicality of the brain is lost in the subjectivity of the self. The inevitable situation that scholars of consciousness studies have to concede is the possibility of the *self-in-the-brain* and *brain-in-the-self*. This is not a simple dualism but an organic dynamism that enables us to go beyond any reductionist theory. We have to begin seeing the brain not just in the vat in the laboratory and the self not just in culture, but also discover the potentialities and the possibilities of the core-self that transcends all binaries. The core-self gives us the possibility to conceptualize a deep, organic self that is not influenced by the physical, mental or social self. The core-self is the space of consciousness in its purest and most inclusive form, from where one gets the courage and bodily adjustments to transcend the challenged psychosomatic identity toward self-healing.

References

Chalmers, D. (1995). The puzzle of conscious experience. *Scientific American, 273*, 62–68.

Crick, F., & Koch, C. (1990). Towards a neurobiological theory of consciousness. *Seminars in Neuroscience, 2*, 263–275.

Humphrey, N. (2006). *Seeing red: A study in consciousness*. Cambridge: The Belknap Press of Harvard University Press.

Merleau-Ponty, M. (1964). *The primacy of perception*. Evanston: Northwestern University Press.

Metzinger, T. (2009). *The ego tunnel: The science of the mind and the myth of the self.* New York: Basic Books.

Varela, F., Thompson, E., & Rosch, E. (1991). *The Embodied Mind: Cognitive Science and Human Experience.* Cambridge: MIT Press.

Chapter 2
Brain and the Self

Human experience is a dance that unfolds in the world and with others. You are not your brain. We are not locked up in a prison of our own ideas and sensations. The phenomenon of consciousness, like that of life itself, is a world-involving dynamic process. We are already at home in the environment. We are out of our heads.

—Alva Noë, 'Out of Our Heads: Why You Are Not Your Brain, and Other Lessons from the Biology of Consciousness', 2009, p. 8

The brain is inarguably the most important organ of the human body studied to understand the working of sensations, emotions and consciousness. The single unit of information and experience that connects sensations and emotions to consciousness is the 'self'. Brain and the self are the common life threads that are used today by neuropsychiatry, neuropharmacology and philosophy to get a conceptual hold on one of the most intractable problems of humankind, namely, 'consciousness'.

Discussion on the self follows two major streams. Self is debated as a cognitive concept that helps find the missing ends between physical and psychological functions. Self is also viewed as the locus of conscious experience. However different the arguments for these two positions are, it is accepted that human behaviours, attitudes and emotions are intricately tied to the discrete neural structures on one side, and the indivisible experiential self on the other.

2.1 Brain's Profile

An average brain weighs about 1,300–1,400 g and accounts for about 2 per cent of the body weight. The human brain has passed through several phases of evolutionary history to reach its present complexity. It took 13,000 years for the skull to

S. Menon, *Brain, Self and Consciousness*, Studies in Neuroscience, Consciousness and Spirituality, DOI: 10.1007/978-81-322-1581-3_2,

grow into the present size. It took 3.5 billion years for the human nervous system to form the present complex specializations. It took a hundred thousand years for humans to have the mental capabilities that we have today.

The human brain contains over 80 billion neurons and many times as many supporting cells. The components of the brain and spinal cord are the 10,000 distinct varieties of neurons, trillions of supportive cells and synaptic connections, about 100 neurochemical regulators and miles of axons and dendrites. Neuronal networks transmit information via synaptic junctions through electrochemical processes and together present a seamless sensory and mental experience.

About 15–20 per cent of the blood flow from the heart is dedicated for the brain. In biological terms, the body enables one's brain with the adequate quantities of oxygen, glucose, minerals and other nutrients, and deprivation of these for more than a few seconds result in unconsciousness or irreversible change in brain functions. Such is the biological profile of the delicate brain. At the same time what makes brain the most complex biological organ is its ability to direct and be influenced by a self and his or her personal experiences. Brain is not a finished organ but flexible for betterment of its structures and functions, and adaptation to new environments and challenges. And this is why it is an 'intelligent' organ that learns through networks built by culture, experiences and new needs.

The classical idea about brain with strictly designated cortical areas and assigned functions is not much in vogue. The view that supersedes is that the brain is a flexible organ with capacities to survive even with less cortical areas. There is growing interest in looking at the brain from a functional perspective than structural, since it is increasingly understood that the brain organizes itself functionally. There are medical cases where patients seem to live 'almost normally' in spite of frontal lobotomy or cortical lesions due to psychiatric conditions (Feinberg 2001). It is suggested that perhaps the limbic system, the seat of emotion, is the most important part of the brain without which normal functioning is impossible (Damasio 1994). There is renewed attention on the subcortical areas of the brain whose roles are still not understood in detail.

The capacity of the brain to switch areas of function when the designated cortical area becomes impaired, termed as neuroplasticity, is finding great interest amongst neuroscientists and philosophers. It is now known that the brain has immense capacity for growth and renewal and its function is modifiable by experience. The synapses change because of new experiences.

The primary output of the brain is experience. In terms of brain function an experience means firing of a cluster of neurons. Firing involves the passage of electrical current away from the cell body down to its axonal length of a neuron. The passage of electric current also activates transference of neurochemicals which function as messengers for the whole body system. Apart from its pervasive electrochemical information system the neural cortex is also structurally divided to integrate different kinds of information. There are different cortical areas that are seemingly demarcated for highly specialized functions. Several brain areas work in unison and harmony to facilitate various sensations. In effect the brain constructs, updates and follows various functional maps.

Several different kinds of topographic maps of the body are stored in the brain cortex, which alter according to new experiences, changing environment and responses. The brain starts forming maps of the body from early in life. With age and experience our brains would have created and stored several complex maps. Brain maps primarily function as bidirectional feedback and feedforward systems. Our experiences change brain maps, and with reorganized maps our experiences also alter. Body maps help us to respond to simple and complex problems whether they are cognitive or affective. Body maps are continuously updated and reorganized as we live our lives. With the change in our physical disposition, life styles, mental attitudes and emotional responses brain maps are updated. We are able to keep track of our movement, position and sense the extremities of the body through the brain maps.

2.2 The Mutual Challenge

Is there a common challenge in brain and self studies that appear over and again? Yes. That is the attempt to explain the unity, continuity, and adherence of our experience, whether it is sensory or mental. To address the unity, adherence and continuity of experience is to address the place of the self in the brain, or the role of the brain in presenting a self.

> One of the most central and important phenomena a theory of consciousness must explain is the sense of unity we have in respect of our conscious mental states. It seems that, for mental representations to be mine, they must, as Kant put it, 'all belong to one self-consciousness'. Indeed, it was just such mental unity to which Descartes appealed in Meditation VI in arguing for the real distinction between mind and body. Whereas the geometrical essence of body guarantees its divisibility, the unity of consciousness ensures that mind is indivisible (Rosenthal 2003, p. 325).

A major challenge to this effort is the fact that, though we tend to commonly address a static unit by calling it 'self', it is a changing phenomenon as a result of our interactions with nature outside (social and biological) and nurture inside (cultural and moral). In the process of its emergence the boundaries of the self seem to change, creating havoc for some (in the case of psychiatric challenges) and peace for others (in the case of spiritual experiences). Where is that self without which we cannot make sense of anything that goes around however physiologically backed up it is? While the skin beautifully covers up all the anatomy and chemistry of a biological system without any spillouts, the self covers up the body too while giving us a feeling of being embodied. Is my self detachable from my body? Is my body inside my self, or is my self inside my body?

We have asked the mind–body question for centuries. But this question becomes even more complex when it comes to the place and function of self. Philosophically, we continue to ask about the mind–body unity—how mind and body, which are qualitatively different, connect and give rise to meaning and purpose of life. The binding problem and the Chalmersian hard problem (Chalmers

1995)[1] showcase the age-old mind–body divide in the context of consciousness. Both demand functional mechanisms and conceptual frameworks for mutual influence. The 'hard problem' is more about a 'mind' than about a 'self'. The 'harder problem' is to delineate the wirings that will tell us how quantitative, discrete, physical, neural processes bind and give rise to qualitative, unitary, subjective conscious experience. In short, how do parts add up and give rise to a sum which is more than the parts put together? The harder problem of consciousness is about the subjectivity of experience.

The 'alter ego' of the brain is known through the person's self. On the one hand the brain is all about its chemistry and cortical structures, and on the other it is about a subtle self that often stays behind, and endures the brain through different experiences. To a great extent the brain influences the way we think and behave. But interestingly, the self in return can influence and reverse engineer behaviour in certain ways. The soft and hard questions on consciousness point to the binding of biochemical mechanisms for a physiological function such as sensation, and to the relevance of such a sensation for the subjective experience of a person. The interconnections between the brain and the self are hence used in neuropsychiatry.

Consciousness is projected by some to be a distinct quality—an emergent product of brain processes (Cabanac et al. 2009). For others all of our personal experiences are reducible to an algorithm, and the brain is a sophisticated computational model (Churchland and Sejnowski 1994). There are also theories that uphold that the majority of the mental processes that control and contribute to our conscious experience happen outside our conscious awareness (Gazzaniga et al. 2002). Another proposal is that all that which constitutes the self can be reduced to the synaptic connections—the neural pathways. To that effect Joseph LeDoux writes:

> People don't come preassembled, but are glued together by life. And each time one of us is constructed, a different result occurs. One reason for this is that we all start out with different sets of genes; another is that we have different experiences. What's interesting about this formulation is not that nature and nurture both contribute to who we are, but that they actually speak the same language. They both ultimately achieve their mental and behavioral effects by shaping the synaptic organization of the brain. The particular patterns of synaptic connections in an individual's brain, and the information encoded by these connections, are the keys to who that person is (LeDoux 2002, p. 3).

Of the many attempts to define the locus of consciousness in the brain, a successful one has been the effort to trace the neural correlates of consciousness (NCC). The NCC approaches serve two functions: (1) to establish identity relations between the neural correlate and the conscious experience; and (2) to find the causal relations between the two. Interestingly, the founders of NCC theory themselves were sceptical about the complete success of the attempt. They wrote:

> Everyone has a rough idea of what is meant by consciousness. We feel that it is better to avoid a precise definition of consciousness because of the dangers of premature definition.

---

[1] See Chaps. 1, 3 (3.2.1) in this volume. Easy problems are problems that relate to physiological processes to explain sensory experiences. Hard problem is how discrete, physical, quantitative processes bind together to give a unitary, subjective and qualitative conscious experience.

> Until we understand the problem much better, any attempt at a formal definition is likely to be either misleading or overly restrictive, or both (p. 264).

2.3 NCC and Unconscious Perceptions

A stronger position to NCC is the replacement of the causal relation between neural correlate and the conscious experience by an identity relation—that there is nothing other than the neural process. The neural process is the conscious experience.

A position that favours functionalism would question the need of consciousness to have sensations and perceptions. Do we need the self to respond to what we perceive? One of the strong proponents of the unconscious processing that happens in the brain is Nicholas Humphrey. He believes that the self is not made entirely of conscious or explicit events. Many perceptual processes are implicit and we are not conscious of them. With his training in primatology, psychology and cognitive science, Humphrey nonchalantly dismisses the subjective nature of consciousness and the ontological reality of self.

In his book, *Seeing Red* (2006), Humphrey investigates the traditional mind-body problem in the context of consciousness. How are conscious experiences related to the physical brain? Adhering to Rylean behaviourism and identity theory,[2] Humphrey suggests that instead of finding a causal explanation for consciousness we need to find the neural correlate for each conscious mental experience. It is to be shown that the NCC is identical with the content of the brain.

Consciousness is nothing other than sensations. We cannot talk about consciousness without sensations. He argues that all perceptions are unconscious and all sensations are actions. According to Humphrey, in the case of seeing a red object, there are two red things—the red object projected and the red sensation (visual experience). The perceiver sees the object, but they do not see the visual experience of the object. They consciously see real things in the real world and not their experiences of those things. Perception of the red object and sensation of it are independent. We have the illusion that sensation and perception are linked because they occur at the same time. Sensation and perception, although they are triggered by the same event, are essentially independent and occur not in series but in parallel, and only interact, if they ever do, much further down the line (Humphrey 2006, p. 50). Visual experience is a form of action. For Humphrey, having a red sensation, waving your hand, and shouting at someone—all the three are actions.

> Consciousness is made of a certain kind of physical activity inside the subject's head. And this activity, we can assume, has been designed by natural selection, using nothing other than the resources of a biologically evolved nervous system (Humphrey 2006, p. 75).

---

[2] Gilbert Ryle criticized the Cartesian mind–body dualism and mocked the notion of the 'ghost in the machine', suggesting that the workings of the mind are not different from bodily acts; rather, they are identical.

Humphrey supports his claim that perceptions are unconscious, with several arguments. In the case of blindsight, some kind of visual perception takes place. But there is no conscious, visual experience. Perception of the object exists without the 'sensation' of seeing. Another example he mentions is that of subliminal perception whereby an advertiser gets a message across so rapidly that we are unconscious of seeing it on the television screen. Just as there can be perception without sensations, there can be changes in sensation without corresponding changes in perception. When a person is under the influence of LSD and other hallucinogens they may have the sensation that a chair has become gigantic while still perceiving the regular chair. The general argument that Humphrey makes is that there are various instances in which the conscious visual experience and the unconscious perception come apart.

One of the best criticisms for Humphrey's position, and the maintenance of the qualitative nature of experience, is given by Searle (2006). Searle considers mind and brain as belonging to different dimensions. Humphrey attempts to place conscious experience and the physical brain in the same space: Mind has qualitative subjectivity. Brain does not have it. The experience of seeing red has a qualitative subjectivity, but the neuron firings that produce this do not have this. Seeing red is a first-person phenomenon. Neuron firings are third-person objective phenomena which look theoretically similar.

2.4 Body and the Conspiracy of Experience

Just because some perceptions can take place without the subject's conscious awareness we cannot conclude that perception is unconscious. Blindsight only suggests that there are several perceptual visual pathways in the brain, and not all of them are conscious. We cannot say that the only form of consciousness one can have is sensation. It is possible that we can have no sensations at all. Consciousness is not seeing alone or just a bunch of sensations. The mystery of consciousness lies in its eluding but ever-present subjective self that reveals through experiences.

Experience is the crux of the problem for both brain sciences and self studies. Relying on self reports one might say that what an experience entails cannot be described clearly and in exhaustive words. But then there are few invariable components and processes that are involved in any experience such as a person, unitary awareness, relevance to past events and future expectations, and essentially a subjective feel of belonging and owning the uniqueness of that experience. Therefore, experience tells us that it is not just 'having a self' but 'being a self'. It makes a tremendous effort to understand, and even before that, to design the methodology, for knowing what is *being a self*.[3] That experience brings with it a person on whom the

[3] For a discussion on 'being a self', see Chap. 9.

content of experience adheres has been a metaphysical problem for classical philosophy in the east and the west. This is demonstrated by the discussions on relations between self, mind and origins of knowledge. While classical traditions have looked at experience with more or less an archived tone, as something that *was there* at some point of time, phenomenological schools focus on lived experience that continue in time primarily because of its embodiment. Phenomenology considers body to be central in requiring the experience to be explained in a diachronic manner. Our experiences have relevance not only in this moment, but also in the subsequent moment. And most importantly, there is continuity and fluidity between the two moments, and it is that which makes experience stick to us in an intimate way.

In the Western world, the significance of the body in conceptualizing and defining the self, inspired by the works of Husserl and Merleau-Ponty, was initiated by Varela et al. (1991). Varela extended the limits of the body from an object to an action. Not only that our mind, cognitions and mental objects are embodied, but also our actions and ensuing capacities are embodied. In the ancient eastern world the views on body have been mostly pluralistic and not overshadowed by metaphysics inorder to establish the non-corporeality of body. Eastern traditions of philosophy and medicine conceptualize body as a generic term, and its specifics known in relation with its situatedness in the respective world.

Embodiment has today become a darling concept for many cognitive scientists and philosophers to ground consciousness (in body) and still retain its transcending power. The liberation sought is for the body that is no more, or not just physical but an intricate representation without which our ability to use language, hold objects, enjoy coffee, love another, be creative and all such potencies become unaffordable. Gibson's concept of 'affordance' (Gibson 1986) has helped cognitive scientists to extend behaviours from the body to an environment, and from non-human animals to the humans. The social brain theorists argue for a social process, distributed across brain, body and the environment, which is responsible for the emergence of consciousness. The incidents of the use of tools in bonobos monkeys have extended the significance of 'social tool use' to 'social cognition'. But if we doubt whether the idea of embodied behaviour is yet another version of behaviourism, at least some respond in the negative.

> … embodied behavior is not a return to *behaviorism*. This is because perception and action form 'oopy structures' where action generates perceptual feedback that, in turn, generates further action, so that outward behavior becomes an important co-contributor to the processes, including neural processes, which generate further behavioral response (Barrett et al. 2007, p. 571).

2.4.1 Why Embodiment?

The physicality of the body is insufficient to explain the complex attributes it possesses, and hence cannot be the common cauldron for containing the elements of transcendence that are non-corporeal. In effect, embodiment is best appreciated in the context of non-embodied consciousness. The concept of the body as well as the experience of the body, even if it is extended beyond its physicality, is limited and will not be able to take the rush of consciousness in the long run. To equate the self with the body, and, the human body with the animal body, might serve a purpose to eliminate the Cartesian substance dualism. But the irony is that 'persons' still survive as organic and unique entities. On the heightened interest in embodiment and body identity theories Shoemaker made a perceptive comment way back in 1999, which is valid today as well. He writes:

> … philosophical enthusiasm for the body has reached such pitch, in recent years, that those who deny that persons are their bodies are likely to find themselves stigmatized as 'Cartesians'.
>
> … whatever else persons are, they are subjects of mental states. And as subjects of mental states, they had better have the persistence conditions that go with this. It had better be the case that when mental states generate their appropriate successor states, or their appropriate behavioral expressions, those successor states belong to the person who had the states that generated them, and those behaviors are on the part of that person (Shoemaker and Strawson 1999, pp. 287, 300).

Let us bring back the question earlier posed: What are the elements in a typical simple experience? To begin with we may question whether any experience can be marked as 'simplistic'. Even seeing a flower, or hearing a sound, or feeling the soft texture of a rose petal, or any such sensation comes with an accompanying barrage of memories, desires, feelings and associated goals. The immediate correlate of experience is a self-sense that inheres in the various components of an experience, and also unites them to give meaning and continuity synchronically and diachronically. A typical experience (such as a visual sensation) involves thoughts, sensations, feelings and moods associated with it and perhaps unique to it. This means that all experiences are already placed in a context and can also invoke new contexts. There is a grand narrative in and around every experience, contributed by the history, dreams and hope of the person.

Any experience is held tight for the experiencer through a self-concept, which at any point gives an idea of who one is, which acts as the conceptual filter, governs habits and behaviours, and also makes self-transcendence possible. What gives relevance to the experience is the experiencer who owns it and is influenced by it. We are able to move from one experience to another, or collate different experiences, and archive them in memories because of the self-concept. To understand self-sense is to also see how the self-concept is continually updated or transformed. Self-concept is fed by the 'me and other' divide we form, the way we reflect upon oneself and the other, and our theory of mind to design our decisions and actions according to the assumptions of what the other mind is going through. The self-sense that we experience every moment and over time is invariably tied to body-sense and a core-self that is not ideated but which presents the possibility to be reflected in various levels and complex depths.

As we explain complex and deep capabilities that humans possess such as pointed reflection, detached watching, enduring calmness and unconditional contentment, the body becomes a poor and insufficient concept to accommodate the onslaught of its possibilities. Even the master trainer the world has seen of the entangled body-mind complex, Patanjali, does not endorse the body, mind, and the body-mind complex to have a lasting ontology. *Samadhi*, the highest state of consciousness, according to Patanjali's yoga, is the tasting of *kevalatva*, the oneness, of pure consciousness. The body mediates experience. The notion of pure consciousness and its non-intentional nature does not fit within the framework of any embodied experience.

2.5 Harder Problem of Experience and the Easy Problem of the Body

The idea of a core-self and its existence have been differently theorized and interpreted by scientists and therapists. I use core-self to mean the deep organic self that is not influenced by the physical, mental or social self. Core-self is a space of consciousness without forms and names and is the source of self-healing. Much of the discussions on body and embodiment have hijacked the possibility and presence of the core-self which is non-embodied and non-ideated. Core-self is not an emergent or minimal entity that is dependent on the body and bodily functions, though it expresses through them.

The larger question that arises from the curious behaviour of the body-sense is twofold. One, what is that sense which recognizes that there is an absence of a body-sense? Second, what is that sense which feels the sensation of the body part which is physically absent? In other words, how or to whom is the sense of the body-absence and the body-sense felt?

Two philosophical problems that arise from a straight jacketed analysis of experience is the inherent subject-object divide, and the amount of the 'other' in 'me', and amount of 'me' in the 'other'. Are the 'other' and 'me' intrinsically different? What stuff are they made of?

We may have an intuitive sense of the other, but it is very difficult to have a clear, articulated description of oneself. The central problem that underlies the first-person nature of consciousness is the entanglement of the body-sense and the self-sense in it. Studies on body-schema and body-image attempt to delineate the body-sense from the self-sense in first person experience. It is important to examine both these senses: are they distinct, and if distinct how? If not, where and how they are entangled? What constitutes these basic, everyday senses?

There are fundamental phenomenological and philosophical questions that are absolutely necessary even to attempt an enquiry into the twilight space where the brain and the self stay in embrace creating a magnificent world of experience. Apart from the basic discipline of philosophy, neurobiology and neuropsychiatry help us to ground questions on matters of experiential concern.

According to the Eastern philosophical tradition of Advaita Vedanta,[4] consciousness is self-luminous. Consciousness not only illuminates an object but is also self-luminous. Both sensation and introspection are available for conscious agents. What Humphrey does not consider is the self-luminous nature of consciousness. In his approach, consciousness is more or less a cognitive function that leads to (visual) sensation. The qualitative nature of consciousness in the form of an experiencing self is not of much consequence according to this theory. What the reductive approaches to explain experience in terms of cognitive functions miss is the flowing, rich nature of the self.

2.6 What is the Self? Can it be Defined by its Characteristics and Functions?

Centuries have passed since the connections between matter and consciousness, the body and the self, have been debated with unflinching vigour but without any clear solution to comprehend the nature of this relation. Any definition of the self has been problematic since historic times.

The discussion on the subjective nature of experience, qualia, stays incomplete without bringing in the role of self. Ramachandran (2003, p. 113) considers qualia and the self as two sides of the same coin though he reduces both to neural processes. Ramachandran, in his five list attributes for self (2003, pp. 113–14) talks about embodiment, agency, and the ability to be self-aware as the important features of self. We have a sense of belonging or ownership to the body. We exercise free will. We self-reflect.

According to Dennett (1989) the self is a ‘non-minimal selfy self’. It is the abstract centre of narrative gravity (Dennett 1991). Strawson (1997) considers self as a cognitive ‘distinctively mental’ phenomenon. Gazzaniga (2006) finds ‘brain's left hemisphere interpreter’ to be responsible for the ‘ongoing narrative of our self-image’. But according to Gallagher (2000) it is a distributed and decentred self. For Damasio (1999), the self is core and autobiographical.

For many developmental psychologists the self is important because it can be situated in the brain. Whether the self is an emergent phenomenon, or is identical with the brain processes, what makes the self interesting is its relation with the brain in order to explain its existence. Cognitive neuroscience has become successful because of its exciting and impossible agenda to understand all human expressions with the help of a biological organ and its

[4] Advaita Vedanta is the philosophical tradition propounded by Adi Sankaracharya in the 8th century AD. According to its epistemology, unlike other objects of experience, ‘consciousness’ does not need another external source of illumination. Consciousness is self-manifest and self-luminous. For further elucidation on this topic, see http://www.iep.utm.edu/adv-veda/.

number and symbol crunching abilities. In short, the project of mainstream trends in cognitive neuroscience is to find how the brain creates the self and its experience.

> Cognitive neuroscience has been driven by the idea that by reductionist analysis of mechanisms within a solitary brain one can best understand how the human mind is constituted and what its nature is. The brain thus came to appear as the creator of the mind and the experienced world (Fuchs 2011, p. 196).

The tendency to biologically situate the self in the brain has faced scepticism. A notable comment is from Shaun Gallagher. He writes:

> The project rather should be what happens in the brain when self-as-subject is engaged in the world, in specific actions and in specific social contexts. This requires not only the sophisticated tools of the neuroimaging lab, and the brilliant experiments of neuropsychology, but also the subtly conceptual tools of philosophy (Gallagher 2011, p. 130).

It is essential to engage with the world to learn about the self not as one other idea but as a living, intimate phenomenon in our experiences. There is a continuity in all our experiences which brings forth the past, present and future at the same moment. In that continuity we experience a unity of discrete psychological phenomena that is presented to us seamlessly, binding our memories, perceptions, cognitions, imagination, emotions and sensations. We are capable of thinking using information from the past and expectations about the future. Memories are closely connected and contiguous to all our experiences. Such continuity is felt adhering to a single unit of consciousness which we call as my-self. Contrary to the Cartesian dictum 'I think, therefore I am', in our daily life we first *are*, and therefore are able to do many things which are mental and physical. Otherwise all our physical and mental acts would not have a place to adhere to and would be floating around. Cartesian dualism is more a theoretical construct to distinguish the complex functions that the human self performs. And the dual and split existence are not experientially true.

If so, what do we understand by 'experience'? The meaning of an experience is the value given to that experience by way of responding to it in terms of a physical and mental action, attitude, emotive valence, memory evoking, consequential thinking and value system, all assimilating to contribute to the perception of purpose. Every experience leaves a mark from the past and carries forward a mark to the future. It is our ability to move forward with identified expectations and plans for future that gives directions to the purpose, and finally making an experience meaningful. Every experience contributes to the purpose of living in body and mind. But the realm of perceiving the purpose and thereby creating a meaning itself need not be a result of sensory and cognitive capabilities but the result of our innate relation with the inner core self that can be identified with a space of possibilities.

We are able to give interconnected meanings to our experiences, learn from our mistakes, form beliefs, cherish hopes, have insecurities, express emotions, reflect upon the faux pas we make in life—all these rich forms of experiences with an unwavering unity and coherence. The first and foremost features of self are being (to put it more experientially, the 'am-ness'), continuity, adherence, coherence and unity. All through these several features of self what runs is that at any point we are capable of different degrees of awareness and reflection. Perhaps in the evolutionary scale what marks the distinctness of the human self is our capacity to be self-aware in multiple, complex and deeper levels. The ability to be self-aware and self-reflect emerges from the 'am-ness' or the 'being' nature of the self. All noble and reified values such as freedom, goodness and health are intricately tied to the 'being' nature of the self, and if well-integrated these contribute to the wellbeing of the individual. *Being* helps the self to self-heal and to lead to its wellbeing.

For all of us, the boundaries of self shift and shrink when challenged by personal, social, emotional, and cultural elements. Spiritual traditions tell us how the smaller, egotistic actor-enjoyer self can be transcended to realize finer planes of consciousness. Self's capability for expansion and non-dual inclusion seems to be vital for Vedantic and similar spiritual traditions. Neuropsychiatry gives us narratives and confabulations of subjects, with brain impairments due to amputations, lesions or psychiatric reasons, who find it hard to stay with a coherent self.[5] Neuropsychology tells us about curious challenges the brain give to the self and the self give to the brain,[6] causing disturbances to our otherwise natural intuition for proprioception—the feeling and knowledge of the position of the body in space. The first acquaintance to the immediate expression of our self, that is our body, itself is presented to as a unified psychophysical whole thanks to many mappings that the brain has devised in collaboration with the feedback received from our daily encounters with the world.

Both neuroscience and spiritual traditions are replete with mind-boggling accounts of challenges and possibilities for the self, literally and figuratively. Both acknowledge the mutual challenge between the body and the spirit, the brain and the self. The conundrum of consciousness continues to stay for the sciences, psychology and philosophy.

Boundaries of self-sense are flexible, contributing to better or worse existences. Nevertheless, that the boundaries shift is no evidence for establishing that there is no self. All the while in and through different experiences an overall value of the self-sense stays that carries forward the agenda of seeking purpose and thereby achieving meaning. Disruption in the body–sense is not tantamount to the absence of a core-self.

Any theory of self will have to also accommodate the wellbeing of the individual so that we never forget that what we theorize is a living, breathing, talking, loving, individual with emotions, and not an automaton who is not subject to the frailties of human living such as love, jealousy, hope and a feeling of collective comradery.

---

[5] For instance, see (Ramachandran and Blakeslee, Phantoms in the Brain 1998).

[6] For instance, see (Lenzenweger 2011, p. 272).

2.7 Agency, Emotions and Altered Self

The flexible nature of the brain is accompanied by the enigma—the self is somehow able to make sense of the neural changes and create corresponding changes in sensations and personal identity. Self-effort, will power, positive thinking, love, compassion, spiritual quietude and such qualities are found to enhance brain functioning in the case of patients who face mental and physical challenges. Until now we have concerned ourselves with the neural correlates of consciousness. The stories of personal strength in coping, role of empathy and altruism, and meditative realms of consciousness, encourage us to find if there are *self-correlates* of consciousness. Self-correlates seem to alter the functions of neural correlates and neural pathways in curious ways.

A fascinating development in brain studies and cognitive sciences in recent time is the alteration in perceptions about reason, its superiority and cognitive closedness. Rationality that is considered as the hallmark of human expression is complemented by the affective face of the individual. How our emotions are felt, expressed and used, will also determine effectiveness in the way we make decisions. Both affective neurosciences and emotion theorists project biological markers of health to be decided by those traits that would favour prosocial behaviour, interpersonal relations, situational mastery, life satisfaction, and discovering meaning and purpose in life.

Mainstream studies in cognitive science focus on reason-driven qualities of consciousness. When even a subject matter such as feeling is studied in an exclusively rational fashion, Damasio's and LeDoux (2002) approach to integrate emotion into the study of self is noteworthy, though the bias is mostly biological. Damasio considers consciousness and emotions as states of the body, more specifically, the immune system. He uses the Cartesian dualism as a point of departure and argues based on neuroscientific research that reason and emotion are closely linked. He distinguishes feelings from emotions (Damasio 1999). Emotion is physical. Feeling is mental. For Damasio, emotions are neural processes that respond to a stimulus. Emotion is the reaction for a stimulus to choose flight-or-fight options. It is also responsible for the homeostatic regulation in the body. Here too a similar question arises as in the case of qualia. If all that is meant by qualia is to automatically provide organisms with survival-oriented behaviours, then why a subjective feel is involved in emotion? Can homeostasis and response to stimulus happen without generating a subjective emotion and an agent who owns it?

Despite the complementing and at times contradicting theories, have we progressed in revealing the mysteries of consciousness? Perhaps we have taken a significant alternate route. The discussion on mind that prevailed in the earlier part of this century is now passed on to the idea of 'self'. To understand the functional nature of consciousness, mind, its cogitations and cognitions are important. But to see through the subjective qualities that consciousness delivers for human experience, self as a whole is to be considered. We all agree that the ultimate puzzle of consciousness is not even the subjective nature of the experience, but the subject itself who seems to weave the beautiful tapestry of rich, colourful, complex experiences.

The recent shift in focus from the mind to the self is accompanied by new trends in biology and psychology. Biology has moved on from the excitement about 'sociobiology' to incorporating counterintuitive ideas, such as empathy, compassion, altruism, and most importantly, emotion. Psychology has marked a detour from the deterministic evaluation rooted in behaviourism, and the repressed, pathological orientation of a patient, to the subjective wellbeing and life satisfaction of a healthy, choice-making individual. And, Libet's experiments (1985) though influenced a few philosophers to make hasty theories about the absence of free will, informed explanations about electrochemical activities that occur in the brain has shown it to the contrary.

2.8 Dual Worlds: Biology and Philosophy

The conceptual questions that the flexible nature of the brain have brought out are twofold. One is more biological and the other philosophical. The biological question is to find out that area of the brain which is indispensable for consciousness without which regeneration of neural cells will not have relevance. The philosophical question brings up the ancient but yet unsolved issue of human identity, and asks if the brain itself is an agent. The progress in science from a 'homunculus'[7] to a 'conscious automatum'[8] to the 'philosophical zombie'[9] to 'single neuron'[10] studies has helplessly carried over the mystery of consciousness to this day. The history of brain studies spans from phrenology to the use of highly sophisticated brain scanning techniques to understand various functions of consciousness. The frustrating but enchanting mystery about consciousness is that every time we find a neural correlate or a new theory, the central concern looms large, which is, how to account for the wholesome subject who owns consciousness. But this does not mean that the eye of the puzzle—consciousness—is an illusion or that it is only a commentary of language or that it cannot be defined at all. To this effect, Damasio writes:

> The argument that consciousness is impossible to define is equally weak. It is certainly true that the definition is not easy and that unless special care is taken to define, at the outset of any investigation or presentation, what is really being meant by the term, a considerable confusion will ensue. In the end, most of us have a sense of what

---

[7] Dennett mockingly describes Descartes' idea of the immaterial soul as the 'homunculus' in his theory of the Cartesian theatre (Dennett 1991).

[8] Thomas Huxley in 1874 suggested that animals (and human beings) are conscious automata, meaning the mind is a product of the neural functions of the body.

[9] A philosophical zombie is a human being bereft of conscious experiences or feelings. It is a common concept in thought experiments in consciousness studies.

[10] Recent studies suggest that single neurons can influence human behaviour and action, contrary to the older belief that it is a collection of neurons that contribute to behaviour. For an elucidation on 'single neuron studies', see http://www.nature.com/news/2007/071219/full/news.2007.392.html.

is meant by consciousness. Most of us, if pressed, produce a definition of consciousness that is patently recorded in the appropriate entry of any quality dictionary: consciousness is that which permits 'awareness of self and surroundings'; or permits 'the awareness of one's own existence, sensations, thoughts, surroundings'. No dictionary fails to present such a definition, usually at the top of the list of definitions (Damasio 1998, p. 1880).

The entangled nature of the brain and the self, its free will, and the enigma of personal uniqueness is the mystery of consciousness, which was likened to the 'unaccountable appearance of the djinn when Alladin rubbed his lamp' by Thomas Huxley,[11] 125 years back. The lamp is the electrochemically complex organ called the brain. The mystery continues not because of the philosopher's adamant metaphysics, but because of the neurologist's advanced techniques that fail to uncover the hidden djiin. The final frontier of consciousness reminds us that the challenging philosophical issues that are at the root of human identity are inconspicuously tied up with the way humans are biologically and culturally endowed.

The Platonic dual world theory, Cartesian mind-body dualism, and the Chalmersian easy problems and the hard problem divide, imply Cartesian dualism and exclusivity of the *res extensa* (that which is extended in space) and *res cogitans* (that which is purely mental). The idea of the body in much of the cognitive science literature is skewed and restricted, being mostly limited to functional representationalism. The Vedantic notion of three bodies (such as the physical, subtle and causal bodies) and embodiment of *Jiva* (the experiential self) breaks through the either-or aporia. For Vedanta the dualist perspective is a transactional tool from the point of view of the body and not a valid one from the point of view of the *Atman* (the pure self). The inside-outside view is from the point of view of the body and not of pure consciousness. This does not mean that the hierarchy is real or that pure consciousness is at the top of the hierarchy. The emphasis is on a subjectivity that is embodied by a liberated person. Embodied liberation, *jivanmukti*, according to Vedanta is centring the body in pure consciousness, and not squeezing consciousness to fit into undersized notions of the body. Vedanta's take on subjectivity retains the somatic expressions of the body, while invoking a 'pure subjectivity', going beyond personal identity which is framed exclusively by life-sustaining bodily functions.

Today, though phenomenology-inspired cognitive sciences have saved the 'body' from being just a tissue-muscle physical thing to something more subjective, cognitive science is still stuck with the notion of a discrete, disconnected, and deconstructed body whose agency is defined around exclusive cognitive functions rather than organismic expressions. And in the process, the brain itself becomes the agent for action. For instance, Galen Strawson describes the project of phenomenology as follows:

The central task of phenomenology, when it comes to the problem of the self, is to analyze the complex, cognitive experience-determining element self that is active in self-experience and that gives it its distinctive character. Once one has determined the content of this experience-structuring element, one can go on to ask the ontological question 'Is there anything in reality to which it applies?'(Strawson 2009, p. 3).

[11] See McGinn, The Mysterious Flame: Conscious Minds in a Material World, 1999, p. 17.

A central concern that arises from the recent interest in perceiving brain as a 'conscious agent' is our very concept of agency and choice-making. Are we confounding the function of a subjective, conscious agent with a biological organ that aids in making decisions and choices?

2.9 Puzzles for Another Decade

The change in perceiving the brain as a biological organ, and human capacities as emergent outpourings of neural processes, poses before us several million-dollar questions: Where and how in the brain is the 'self' housed? How does the self make adaptive changes in one's personality corresponding to the changes in the brain? How does the self influence and alter neurochemical functions of the brain? How is that we can verbalize and report our internal states through self-reflection and introspection? How does the brain integrate information from physiological and mental sources in order to control behaviour and inner states? Can the brain address its structural and functional challenges without the recourse to the self? Can there be a self without the interface of the brain and the limbic system? Are the brain and self constantly challenging each other? How does the brain and the self together create subjective experience? In other words, how does the brain and self conceive their role-play and create the conspiracy of experience where the physicality of the brain is lost in the subjectivity of the self?

These and similar questions may not give immediate answers considering the complex ways in which both our brain and self are cross-wired. They are difficult to answer also because we are yet to design better philosophical conceptual frameworks that are conducive to scientific reductionism as well as humanism. There are fewer consensuses in including the subject and the object, the first-person and the third-person data in a manner that is inclusive. Several medical cases studied by neuropsychiatrists show that the way the patient behaves before and after a cure is not even amenable to arrive at straightforward causal relations between the brain and the self. The subject-object distinction itself is shadowed when the brain behaves in ways not true to its essential physical neural structure. Can the brain be described as distinctly objective and physical when it defies the laws of medicine? How does subjectivity intervene into the predictable physical behaviours of the brain and create medical miracles?

When David Chalmers published the fascinating puzzle of conscious experience and showcased the 'hard problem' of consciousness in the late nineties, little did we realize that the mystery will only double in another decade. Today, with path-breaking studies in neurology, neuropsychiatry, neuropharmacology, and brain scanning techniques, we have covered more distance, and moved further from the puzzle of the conscious experience to the mystery of the self who interplays with brain to facilitate an experiencer, a person in all her glory. The self is the 'harder problem' for the next decade, and perhaps for a distant future. The greatest challenge is to trace the route of the passage, if any, from the brain to the self and its trajectories.

The 'harder problem' is to trace the ways in which the brain challenges the self, and the self challenges the brain. To understand the brain is to gain access to the inherently private and subjective space of the self. It is important to continue the classic mind-body debates that favour functional identity and dualism. But equally significant is to understand the emergence and the placement of the self in the context of an evolving brain which has the capacity to change and adapt. Greater insights into the nature of the self—neural and ontological—will arrive if we focus our research on the challenges that the brain and the self give each other. The brain and the self are the final frontiers of consciousness, not as independent puzzles, but as complexly cross-wired phenomena that will persist to stay magical for human imagination. We will have to wait for the day when the door that intermediates the physical world and the personal world opens and let us in, to appreciate the twilight space with better sight and insight.

References

Barrett, L., Henzi, P., & Rendall, D. (2007). Social brains, simple minds: Does social complexity really require cognitive complexity? *Philosophical Transactions of the Royal Society: Biological Sciences: Social Intelligence: From Brain to Culture, 362*(1480), 561–575.

Cabanac, M., Cabanac, A. J., & Parent, A. (2009). The emergence of consciousness in phylogeny. *Behavioural Brain Research, 198*, 267–272.

Chalmers, D. (1995). The puzzle of conscious experience. *Scientific American, 273*, 62–68.

Churchland, P. S., & Sejnowski, T. J. (1994). *The computational brain.* : A Bradford Book.

Damasio, A. (1994). *Descartes' error: Emotion, reason and the human brain.* New York: G.P. Putnam' Sons.

Damasio, A. R. (1998). Investigating the biology of consciousness. *Philosophical transactions: Biological sciences—the conscious brain: Abnormal and normal, 353*(1377), 1879–1882.

Damasio, A. (1999). *Feeling of what happens: Body and emotion in the making of consciousness.* London: Heinemann.

Dennett, D. (1989). *Cogito, 3*, 163–173

Dennett, D. (1991). *Consciousness explained.* London: Allen Lane.

Feinberg, T. E. (2001). *Altered egos: How the brain creates the self.* Oxford: Oxford University Press.

Fuchs, T. (2011). The brain: A mediating organ. *Journal of Consciousness Studies, 18*(7–8), 196–221.

Gallagher, S. (2000). Philosophical conceptions of the self: Implications for cognitive science. *Trends in the Cognitive Sciences, 4*(1), 14–21.

Gallagher, S. (Ed.). (2011). *The Oxford handbook of the self.* Oxford: Oxford University Press.

Gazzaniga, M. (2006). *The ethical brain: The science of our moral dilemmas.* : HarperCollins.

Gazzaniga, M., Ivry, R. B., & Mangun, G. R. (2002). *Cognitive neuroscience: The biology of the mind.* New York: W.W. Norton & Company.

Gibson, J. J. (1986). The ecological approach to visual perception. Routledge.

Humphrey, N. (2006). *Seeing red: A study in consciousness.* : The Belknap Press of Harvard University Press.

Libet, B. (1985). Unconscious cerebral initiative and the role of conscious will in voluntary action. Behavioral and Brain Sciences, 8(4), 529–539.

LeDoux, J. (2002). *Synaptic self: How our brains become who we are.* New York: Penguin Books.

Lenzenweger, M. F. (2011). *Schizotypy and schizophrenia: The view from experimental psychopathology*. New York: Guilford Press.
Ramachandran, V. (2003). *The emerging mind*. London: The BBC in association with Profile Books Ltd.
Ramachandran, V., & Blakeslee, S. (1998). *Phantoms in the Brain*. New York: William Morrow
Rosenthal, D. M. (2003). Unity of consciousness and the self. *Proceedings of the Aristotelian Society, New Series, 103*, 325–352.
Searle, J. R. (2006). Minding the brain. The New York Review of Books, New York, LIII, 17, 51–55.
Shoemaker, S., & Strawson, G. (1999). Self and body. *Proceedings of the Aristotelian Society, Supplementary Volumes, 73*, 287–332.
Strawson, G. (1997). The self. *Journal of Consciousness Studies, 4*(5–6), 405–428.
Strawson, G. (2009). *Selves: An essay in revisionary metaphysics*. Oxford: Clarendon Press.
Varela, F., Thompson, E., & Rosch, E. (1991). *The embodied mind: Cognitive science and human experience*. Cambridge, MA: MIT Press.

Chapter 3
Beginnings: Biological and Philosophical Accounts of Consciousness

To confine oneself to studying consciousness as such means to consider the phenomenal content of one's mental representations—that is, how they feel to you from the first-person perspective, what it is like (subjectively, privately, inwardly) to have them.

—Thomas Metzinger, 'The Ego Tunnel', (2009), p. 10

Be it the sensation of lingering aroma from the steaming cup of coffee or the choking ache felt at the sight of a homeless in the street, our experiences are intricately wired. The history of consciousness is in fact the history of the making of our experiences. More than the physiology, it is the frailties and sensitivities of humanity that influence our selfhood.

How did consciousness become sophisticated from directing rudimentary visual, tactile, and such other sensations to the grand presentation of a refined sensitive person? What did it entail for consciousness to emerge from a few complex biochemical molecules, electrical impulses and some hundred receptors? Or is consciousness an emergent phenomenon at all? How did developmental and structural changes of the brain plan for the evolution of sensations and feelings through natural selection? Did language and other expressions of culture play a significant role in the transformation of the Homo erectus to the Homo sapiens?

Consciousness has both natural and cultural histories. How over millennia a seemingly simple organ with similar set of brain molecules, neurotransmitters and synapses across insects, fishes, reptiles, birds and mammals led to the emergence of a superior capability called consciousness in humans is a question that has persisted for many centuries. One conjecture is that the relative increase in the size of the human brain and its structural localizations dedicated for monitoring different functions led to the emergence of discrete behaviours, and cognitive functions. The development of neocortex led to better intelligence in terms of fore-planning, decision making and consequential thinking.

The two disciplines that watch brain sciences with interest are primatology and developmental psychology. Both these disciplines believe in the evolutionary

S. Menon, *Brain, Self and Consciousness*, Studies in Neuroscience, Consciousness and Spirituality, DOI: 10.1007/978-81-322-1581-3_3,

origin and development of brain. In general, primatologists would bring in natural evolution and social cognition to explain the behaviour in non-human primates. Probable questions to a primatologist are 'what is an experience' and 'what is a subject' in non-human primates. While there is sparse reference to the concept of self-awareness and ability to reflect, the crux of the theories lies in theories of a variety of social cognition and associated behaviours. In social cognitive approaches, the self is a schema or a grand collection of several schemas.

> The self in this view is a schema or set of schemas which includes abstract semantic knowledge as well as specific episodic memories and may have hierarchical organization like other schemas or concepts (such as "bird," which has nested within it many subtypes; similarly the self has many subcategories). The evidentiary basis for this view is an increasingly large body of literature documenting the role of self-schemas in information processing (Westen 1992, p. 3).

Is the concept of a 'social brain' used to explain a wide variety of human and non-human primate behaviours overrated with sidelined 'anthropocentric commitments' on one side, and dependence on information processing theories on the other? Some recent views imply that social complexity may not need an equivalent degree of cognitive complexity, and that the focus has to shift from exclusive attention on a 'theory of mind' to distributed and embodied cognition. For example, Barrett et al. write:

> The social brain hypothesis is a well-accepted and well-supported evolutionary theory of enlarged brain size in the non-human primates. Nevertheless, it tends to emphasize an anthropocentric view of social life and cognition. This often leads to confusion between ultimate and proximate mechanisms, and an over-reliance on a Cartesian, narratively structured view of the mind and social life, which in turn lead to views of social complexity that are congenial to our views of ourselves, rather than necessarily representative of primate social worlds.... greater attention to embodied and distributed theories of cognition, which get us away from current fixations on 'theory of mind' and other high-level anthropocentric constructions, and allow for the generation of testable hypotheses that combine neurobiology, psychology and behaviour in a mutually reinforcing manner. (Barrett et al. 2007, p. 561).

It is extremely difficult to envisage in non-human primates a similar discussion of the self and consciousness as presented in the human. Certainly the role, and the development, of brain and neural structures is a question that pervades investigation of consciousness in humans and other animals, plants and other life forms.

Brain is evidently a major area for investigation to understand human nature, experience and behaviour, which collectively contributes to consciousness. What rates brain a superior organ of the human body is its incredible complexity and its significant influence on human experiences. Some part or the other of the brain controls and facilitates every movement, thought, sensation, and emotion that we possess.

Brain sciences have faced several changes in fundamental perspectives in the past few decades. Primarily these changes are due to the accommodation of the qualitative expressions of the neuronal brain and bringing them under a neuropsychological purview. Brain research has migrated from the peripheries of biology and psychology to assume a central position within those disciplines. Today, the multidiscipline of neuroscience that emerged from this process ranges from genes to cognition, from molecules to minds (Kandel and Squire 2000).

Methods to understand brain and its mechanisms range from the classical phrenological studies on one end to physiognomy, brain-mapping, neuropsychiatry and neurotheology on the other. The goals vary mostly with scientific specificities. The common ground for the recognition of varied methods and perspectives, which is also a converging response, is the challenge implied by the persistent qualitative characteristic of the brain, namely, its self-orientation. The cases of synesthetes, epileptics, and those who are neurally impaired pose a larger question of the 'owner' of their consciousness—a self.

3.1 Brain and its Functions

An average brain weighs about 1,300–1,400 g and accounts for 2 % of the body weight. It took 13,000 years for the skull to grow into the present size. It took three and a half billion years for the human nervous system to develop. It took a hundred thousand years for humans to have their present mental capabilities.

The components of the brain and spinal cord are the 10,000 distinct varieties of neurons, trillions of supportive cells such as glia cells, and synaptic connections, about a hundred neurochemical regulators and miles of axons and dendrites. They work together to present a seamless sensory and mental experience.

Three major areas form the brain—the cerebral cortex, subcortical structures and the brain stem. The brain has distinct cortical structures and each structure works in unison with other structures, and as a whole. The cortical and sub-cortical structures together enable the brain to channel, interpret, and respond to the information received at the neural pathways. The several widely separated areas of the cortex act simultaneously when a mental task is performed. These areas are dedicated toward specialized functions as well as contribute to the global processes of the brain.

> Although much evidence exists for both localization of functions and for global processes, conflicts in interpreting this evidence have given rise to long-standing controversies in brain science. To explain brain function, "localizationists" favor specificity of local brain modules where as "holists" stress global integration, mass action and Gestalt phenomena (Edelman 1998, p. 49).

There are two theories on the working of the brain, that it is localized and that it is globally integrated. While some areas of the brain are dedicated for certain functions, much of the brain activity resorts to information received in various parts of the brain and processed therein for a final integrated perception or sensation.

3.1.1 *Neuronal Connections*

The average human brain is estimated to have close to 80 billion neurons. Each neuron has parts such as dendrites, an axon and a synapse. Dendrites and axons are specialized extensions of neurons. Dendrites are threadlike extensions that grow out of neurons and bring information to the cell body. Axons take information away from the cell body. Synapse is a specialized structure and is a connection that is caused by an electrochemical process between two neuronal ends. A synapse consists of a presynaptic ending that contains neurotransmitters, mitochondria and other cell organelles; a postsynaptic ending that contains receptor sites for neurotransmitters; and, a synaptic space between the presynaptic and postsynaptic endings. It is across the synapse that information from one neuron flows to another neuron.The billions of neural cells and their synaptic connections together regulate the body, enable learning from a lifetime of experiences, and recall memories and thoughts unique to each one of us.

Neurons vary in shape and size. The size of their cell bodies ranges from four microns to hundred microns. Neurons are similar to other living cells. But they are also unique since they come in varied shapes and also form synaptic connections between each other. The widely popularized theory is that brain cannot replace dead neurons and that the number of neurons stays same for the entire life, and might even become fewer as we age. This theory has been challenged lately and neurologists have reported neurogenesis in adult human brains. Peter Eriksson and his colleagues from Sahlgrenska University Hospital in Sweden, and Fred H. Gage from The Salk Institute for Biological Studies demonstrated that neurogenesis occurs in the brains of adult humans as old as 72 years of age (Eriksson et al. 1998). Production of new neurons, due to neural stem cells (cells that are able to differentiate into many different types of neurons), were cited in the hippocampus, the seat of new learning and memory. Their studies also established that human hippocampus retains its ability to generate neurons throughout life.

This means our brains have the capacity to support lifelong learning given appropriate circumstances. Neurons can form new connections as long as the cells stay healthy. Connections remain at a peak from an age of 4 to 10 years. During these years a child's brain has many more connections than does an adult's brain and uses twice the amount of energy. The more the number of neuronal connections, the better will be the functioning of the brain. The neuronal connections are decided by the inherited growth patterns, response to stimuli including internal stimuli triggered by imagination, new learning, habits and attitudes, personal values, etc.

The basis of the communication between neurons is an electrochemical process. The body receives information through the primary sensations and encodes it as nerve impulses. The movement of messenger chemicals called neurotransmitters facilitates the neuronal communication across the synaptic gap. Neurotransmitters are chemicals that allow the movement of information from one neuron across the synaptic gap to the adjacent neuron. When electrical impulses reach the brain the respective cortical area triggers the release of neurotransmitters which in turn induce electrical impulses travelling from one neuron to another, finally producing a bodily response.

The chemicals in our body such as charged sodium, potassium and chloride ions move in and out of neurons and establish an electrical current. The release of neurotransmitters from the neuron is controlled by the depolarization-hyperpolarization mechanism. The electrical reaction facilitates the release of the neurotransmitter and its movement across the synaptic gap. Neurotransmitters are released from the terminal area in response to an action potential signal. The released neurotransmitter is recognized by a receptor (a peptide) on the adjacent neuron. The reception of the neurotransmitter is followed by a biological effect and a change in the action potential. Once the binding process is complete, the ability of the neurotransmitter to stimulate the biological effect is lost. The receptor then becomes ready to receive another neurotransmitter. Once it reaches the post-synaptic ending the neurotransmitters break down (like acetylcholine), reabsorbed into the terminal region, or diffuse away (like dopamine) from their targeted synaptic junctions. They are eliminated from the body en route the kidneys.

All neurotransmitters cannot bind with all receptors. There is a selective process that decides the binding. The binding is specific and has to fit like a key fits into a lock. Some neurotransmitters activate neurons and others inhibit them. They have different effects depending upon which receptor to which they bind. The abnormalities in the production or functioning of neurotransmitters have been recognized in a number of diseases such as Parkinson's disease, schizophrenia, depression, mood disorders etc. Drugs, alcohol, and caffeine, are known to alter the release and transmission of neurotransmitters.

3.2 Cerebral Cortex and the Four Lobes

The cerebral cortex is the cerebrum's outermost layer which is visible. Below the cerebral cortex are the different subcortical structures. The cerebral cortex is about 3.2 mm thick in human brains, and is highly convoluted. The convoluted structure helps to increase the surface area of the brain without corresponding increase in volume and size. In humans the cerebral cortex accounts for about 76 % of the brain's volume. The six-layered surface of the cortex covers the surface of the cerebrum and goes down into the fissures. Cells in different regions of the cortex coordinate vision, hearing, touch, sense of balance, movement, emotional responses and cognitive functions.

The cerebral cortex is also called the neocortex, being the most recently evolved region of the brain. The neocortex has contributed immensely for the development of human nature characterized by culture, art, science and technologies. It is the newer portion of the brain which is the centre of higher mental functions for humans. With some 80 billion cells, each with 1,000–10,000 synapses and roughly 100 million metres of wiring, the neocortex performs most of the brain's higher cognitive functions. These include sensory perception, generation of motor commands, spatial reasoning, conscious thought, and language use. The various processing centres of the neocortex technically called 'association areas' assemble and decipher neural impulse into meaningful perceptions. By being the centre of sensory and motor control, in a limited sense, we could say that the neocortex has a prominent role in contributing to the experience of 'self'.

According to another prominent anatomical method the brain can be divided down the middle into two hemispheres, the left and the right. The hemispheres are connected by a band of neural fibres called corpus callosum, which passes information from one hemisphere to the other. The respective half of the brain controls the muscle movements of that side. Functioning contralaterally, in an opposite direction, the left side of the cerebrum takes care of the right side of the body and conversely. But most of the functions we perform involve both parts of the brain.

Based on the overlying bone structure, the hemispheres are divided into four lobes: (1) frontal (2) parietal (3) temporal, and, (4) occipital. Different areas of the four lobes process sensory information or coordinate motor output necessary for the control of movement. Of these areas some regions are more directly involved than others with sensory or motor processing. In the order of direct function these areas are divided into primary, secondary and tertiary sensory or motor areas.

The frontal lobe is located in the front part of the cerebrum and handles the functions of planning, emotions, and parts of speech. The frontal lobes have been referred to as the "senior executive" of the brain and personality (Joseph 1990, p. 183). They are associated with goal formation, long-term planning skills, the ability to consider multiple alternatives and outcomes simultaneously, as well as the search and retrieval of memory. The interventions through the frontal lobes can inhibit, suppress, or enhance perceptual and information processing, including learning and memory, through inhibitory and excitatory influences directed to the thalamus, brainstem, or the different lobes of the brain. The frontal lobes are provided with multiple streams of input since they are interlocked with the thalamus, limbic system, brainstem, and the parietal, occipital, and temporal lobes. They are constantly informed about the processing which takes place in other regions of the brain.

The parietal lobe is located above the occipital lobe and behind the frontal lobe. It controls information related to touch, temperature, pain, and pressure and coordinates sensory information. Damage to this area results in difficulties with coordination and movement. The temporal lobe located on the side of the cerebrum contains the primary auditory cortex. It interprets auditory data and contributes to speech and memory functions. The temporal lobes contain the core structures of the limbic system, amygdala and hippocampus and stores spatial, verbal and personal memories. The functioning of the temporal lobe is central to one's personal and emotional identity. Stimulation of the temporal lobe can result in intense auditory or visual hallucinations. The occipital lobe is located behind and below the parietal and temporal lobes. It contains the primary visual cortex that controls the vision system.

3.2.1 Subcortical Structures

There are many specialized areas below the surface of the cortex and are grouped using a division guided by developmental biology such as the forebrain (prosencephalon), midbrain (mesencephalon) and hindbrain (rhombencephalon). The division of the brain into three parts and the study of its structural development have advanced with progress in neuroimaging, behavioural neurology and molecular genetics. Particularly, the understanding of developmental disorders that affect the midbrain and the hindbrain have shed new light in studying mental retardation and autism since malformations of the brain stem and cerebellum often occur as the only recognized malformation in these individuals (Barkovich et al. 2009).

The forebrain (apart from the cerebrum) consists of the basal ganglia, limbic system, thalamus and hypothalamus. Tectum and tegmentum make up the midbrain and is concerned with eye movement, localization of objects and control of movement in general. The hindbrain consists of the cerebellum, reticular formations, pons and medulla oblongata, and are largely devoted to involuntary life-support systems such as heart rate and blood pressure, respiratory and digestive functions. It also controls the coordination and integration of visual information with movement. The brain stem is the core part of the spinal cord that enters the cerebrum and extends up to the hypothalamus. The common representation of brain stem includes pons, midbrain and medulla oblongata. The nerve connections of the motor and sensory systems from the main part of the brain to the rest of the body pass through the brain stem.

The basal ganglia are a collection of nuclei placed in the white matter of cerebral cortex. Basal ganglia and cerebellum together modify movement on a minute-to-minute basis. The motor cortex sends information to both basal ganglia and cerebellum, and both structures send information back to cortex via the thalamus. The output of the cerebellum is excitatory, while the basal ganglia are inhibitory. The balance between these two systems maintains smooth and coordinated movement. The dysfunctions in either systems cause movement disorders such as Parkinson's disease and Huntington's disease.

The limbic system works in an interactive fashion and includes the amygdala, hippocampus, hypothalamus, olfactory cortex, thalamus and other structures such as anterior cingulate gyrus, fornix, septal nuclei etc. The amygdala receives inputs, highly processed information, from the association areas of visual, auditory, and somatosensory cortices. With extensive interconnections with the frontal cortex, its outputs involve arousal, control of autonomic responses associated with fear (fight or flight—aggressive or defensive behaviour), emotional responses and hormonal secretions. The hippocampus—responsible largely for memory and learning—is devoted to formation of new declarative memories and interacts with the temporal lobe to create event memories.

The thalamus is the gatekeeper which keeps a continuous watch on the sensory information that gets into the cerebral cortex. It receives information from visual, auditory systems, spinal cord and relays information to the cerebral cortex. The major function of thalamus is sustaining waking consciousness. Hypothalamus is located below the thalamus and maintains homeostasis. It produces sex, stress and growth hormones and controls basic functions such as blood pressure, body temperature, metabolism, adrenaline levels, sleep-awake pattern, sexual behaviour, body weight and appetite. Another subcortical structure called pons also contributes to the regulation of sleep, feeding and facial expressions.

The cerebellum is called the "little brain" since it has a structure, similar to the cerebrum, with the grey and white matter and cortical folds. Structurally, the cerebellum is also a collection of nuclei, apart from three peduncles (stalks) and a specialized layer of cells called purkinje cells. The purkinje cells are concerned with the coordination of movement. Purkinje cells are affected by diseases and dysfunctions due to toxic exposure (such as alcohol), autoimmune diseases (like vertigo and vestibular imbalance) and genetic mutations (like autism). Purkinje cells release a neurotransmitter called GABA (gamma-Aminobutyric acid) which exerts inhibitory actions on certain neurons enabling them to regulate and coordinate motor movements. The proprioceptive feedback received from the limbs and the motor cortex is compared and movement is corrected accordingly by the cerebellum. The cerebellum is also partly responsible for motor learning, such as riding a bicycle. The dysfunctions of cerebellum mainly contribute to the general inability to determine space and distance, maintain balance, and control movement.

3.2.2 Sensory Processing and Association Areas

The body environment communication happens with the help of interactions between the nervous, endocrine and immune systems. The nervous system is particularly important since it innervates the glands and muscles through various information pathways. The information received from the rest of the body is processed in the brain. Sensory information received from the raw data from the senses is processed by the brain to result in the final presentation of multidimensional and multisensory perceptions. Newberg et al. (2001) state that in the first level of processing the primary receptive areas dedicated to each of the five sensory systems receives raw data and assemble them into preliminary perceptions. In the second level, secondary receptive areas for each of the sensory system further refines the preliminary perceptions. In the third level of processing these perceptions move to association areas. The most sophisticated processing happens in the association areas.

The 'association areas' (apart from sensory and motor areas) are specialized areas, located in the cerebral cortex.There are several association areas of which the major ones are enumerated by Newberg et al. (2001), according to their function, as visual, orientation, attention and verbal conceptual association areas. Association areas are structural regions of the neocortex, that receives inputs from five sensory systems, combines these inputs, and associate them to a meaningful context of memory, emotion and other specificities of experience thereby juxtaposing the experiencing self with the world outside. These regions lie outside the primary, secondary and tertiary, sensory and motor areas.

Orientation association area is situated in the posterior superior region of the parietal lobe, receives inputs mainly from touch, vision and auditory systems, and has multiple connections with the limbic system. Its function is to orient and locate the individual in physical space, judge distances and angles, and safely negotiate a pathway. The left orientation area enables the judgment between objects that can be grasped and objects that are beyond grasp (Newberg et al. 2001). This area plays a greater role in the distinction of the self and the other in our experiences (Joseph 1990). Visual association area presents what is seen in a meaningful context of emotion and memory. Damage to this area takes away the context of the seen object. In blindsight, for instance, serious damage to the primary visual association area prevents visual input from reaching the secondary level. Still, the brain unconsciously recognizes visual data but is unable to associate it with a personal context or specificities. Other instances are Capgras and Cotard's syndromes (Ramachandran and Blakeslee 1998). Attention association area is the pre-frontal cortex which governs all logical and goal-oriented functions apart from the muscular movements. It is described as the 'neurological seat of will' (Joseph 1990). Inabilities in forming goals and intentions, lack of will, and emotional absence, are resultant of damage to this area. Verbal conceptual association area is located at the junction of temporal, parietal, and occipital lobes. This area is responsible for causal thinking, formation of abstract concepts, high order language, and logical functions.

The parietal-temporal-occipital association cortex occupies the interface of the three lobes. It is concerned with higher perceptual functions related to physical sensations, hearing and vision. Complex perceptions are formed by the combination of information from these three sensory systems. The prefrontal association cortex lies on the rostral part of the frontal lobe. This area is crucial for the planning of voluntary movement. The limbic association cortex is located on the medial and inferior surfaces of the cerebral hemispheres of the parietal temporal and frontal lobes and is concerned with motivation, emotion, and memory. Information from various parts of the brain are received and integrated at the association areas to produce multisensory meaningful perceptions within a cognitive and emotional context. This is also made possible by the connection of the association areas with the brain centres of emotion and memory. Association areas are neurally responsible for the subjective nature of human perceptions. Newberg writes:

> … the two sides of the orientation association area are able to weave raw sensory data into the vivid, complex perception of a self and into a world in which that self can move. The fact that this 'self' is not a mental representation, and that it is assembled from bits of raw sensory data, does not mean, of course, that the physical body or the world around it does not exist. The point is that the only way the mind can know the self, and experience the difference between the self and the rest of reality, is through the elaborate, restless efforts of the brain (Newberg et al. 2001, p. 29).

Perhaps because of the relation with the key experiences in our daily lives, disruptions in association areas cause major alterations in the sensory experience often stripping of the psychological meaning, interpretation and context of the personal experience. Essentially, much of neurology and behavioural neurology tells us how much what we call as the experiential self and its consciousness is dependent on the smooth functioning of the brain and its specialized areas. The fundamental principle of neurology is established on the view that what we think of as reality is only a rendition of reality that is created by the brain (Newberg et al. 2001, p. 35) and that consciousness can be understood as a product of evolution through natural selection.

3.3 Body-Mind and Body-Self Debates

The varied expressions of our minds and bodies necessarily involve complex brain activities. But do all life expressions, and the central mark of life, that is consciousness, owe their existence completely to neural mechanisms? The response involves not just the neurosciences, but also philosophy and ethics.

That consciousness is the intrinsic nature of a knowing, feeling, free subject in contrast to an inert deterministic object, is a view that prevailed in the philosophy of the Upanishads[1] and the ancient Greece. Plato identified mind with the head because of its symmetrical structure, and Aristotle to the heart. Western and eastern worlds recognized parallel positions of a single unitary consciousness, as well as a mind that is independent of the body.

In the classical Cartesian case of mind-body dualism the entity of mind represents not just mental functions but also higher capabilities of consciousness such as reflection ('cogito'). Any act of thinking, according to Descartes (1596–1650), suggests the presence of a conscious thinker. Descartes' distinction of mind from the body was deliberate given the influence of scientific revolution caused by Newtonian mechanics in the seventeenth century. Over the preponderance of empirical knowledge guided by sensory information, Descartes suggested mind as an independent source of knowledge and body as a conscious automaton. Consciousness was then a phenomenon riddled with mysticism and unrecognized by science. Yet the basic tenet of dualism was successful to bring into question traces of a self-identity and personhood that possess reflective capacities, along with the lingering puzzle of the interaction between the mind and the body, between the extended material substance and the non-extended, non-local mind.

Hume (1711–1776) rejected the Cartesian view through his 'bundle theory'. He stated that through inner experience one can only identify a variety of discrete experiences and not a single metaphysical entity that remains the same. There is no essential self which is bereft of discrete perceptions. With his penchant for the positivistic framework, Hume suggested that relations between the mind and the body, and the assemblage of discrete percepts are united by two associative principles such as 'association' and 'causation'. Yet, he considered association not as a necessary condition for the mind to exist as one entity, because the mind's percepts can also exist 'unowned' (Patten 1976, p. 68).

---

[1] Upanishads are ancient Indian philosophical texts from circa 4th century BC.

Was Hume right in his concept of the self all the while admitting existence for perceptions? Was he admitting a phenomenology without a self to experience?

> Hume's argument against a substantial ego is based on an important phenomenological fact: the only things we find within interior consciousness are 'perceptions', by which Hume meant all contents of consciousness, including thoughts, desires, feelings, images, sensations, and sense impressions. However, this phenomenological fact is not sufficient to establish Hume's conclusion that there is no substantial ego at the centre of consciousness. It might be the case that the ego is a substance but is inherently unable to cognize itself as such (Washburn 2012, p. 197).

Kant (1724–1804) argued against the Humean position and suggested that the unity and identity of self-consciousness are essential for any form of thought to manifest. He identified apperception as the source of unity in experience, which enables us to have self-reference for any representation. Perhaps Kant foresaw the theory of intentionality which was introduced by Franz Brentano in the nineteenth century. That all of our experiences are intentionally directed sets the possibility of direct introspection as a phenomenological method for both conscious and unconscious mental states.

Kant's postulate of the noumenon and Freud's theory of the unconscious belong to two different systems; however, both proclaim the inherent contradiction in our lives and the aspiration for a free consciousness. Freud argued that humans are subject to unconscious activities and thus subject to a form of natural determinism. But the ego is endowed with a rational faculty that provides the means of both understanding the deterministic forces of the unconscious as well as freeing the ego from their authority. According to Tauber (2009), psychoanalysis depends on an implicit notion of autonomy, whereby the interpretative faculty would free the analysand from the tyranny of the unconscious in order to pursue the potential of human creativity and freedom.

The psychoanalytic self is a self with many representations and often in conflict, which also explains the position that explains psychopathology according to psychoanalytic theories.

> If one were to synthesize the dimensions common to these various psychoanalytic approaches to the self, several common denominators stand out. First, self-representations are seen as multidimensional: A person has a large repertoire of enduring representations that can be quite contradictory, and these representations are encoded in semantic as well as sensory modes (such as images, sounds, smells, etc.). Second, self-representations are affectively laden. Indeed, in most object relations theories the earliest representations are seen as organized strictly along affective lines (e.g., good me, bad me, good mother, bad mother). Third, self-representations are seen as integral components of representational units, which typically involve self-in-relation-to-other. Fourth, representations are assumed to have conscious and unconscious components. Conscious representations are not seen as necessarily similar to their unconscious counterparts, even when both are currently active. A narcissistic patient may, for example, be insisting that he is better than all his superiors precisely because unconsciously he feels weak and inferior. Finally, representations are understood in relation to other representations and to wishes and fears. A person is assumed to have many conflicting representations, and often to fear precisely the same experiences represented in wishes (such as self outdoing father in the tragic-hero

> example). This can be expected to lead to behavior and affects that reflect the person's competing valuations of the self-experience represented (Westen 1992, p. 3).

It is interesting to also take a brief glance at the concept of the self of postmodernist thinkers. Almost all of postmodernism rejects a sensible self that is coherent and continuous. In fact, according to postmodernist thinkers, the self is multitudinous, created by different contexts of social origin, and hence cannot be recreated. On the perishing selves of the postmodernists, a recent reviewer of the concept of ego writes:

> According to postmodernists, the multiplicity and fragmentation of the self are such that the self can never be shaped into a coherently unified whole. In emphatic disagreement with Sartre's notions of the fundamental project and free self-creation, postmodernists insist that our self-authoring abilities are extremely limited. The components of the self are resistant to efforts to unify them not only because they are so great in number and so changingly, obscurely, and conflictingly interrelated but also because many of them are irrecoverably embedded in their social sources and origins. For postmodernists, there is no unified self of any sort, not even a coherently unified ego identity or self-representation. Postmodernists believe that the notion of a unified self is a fiction that veils the inherently plural, protean, embedded, and unself-contained nature of the self (Washburn 2012, p. 213).

In Kant, Freud (psychoanalytic traditions) and in postmodernist thinkers we see the inherent tension between the two forces that build human consciousness: the body and its emergent outcomes that are determined by the laws of nature; and reason which is 'practical' which can liberate the mind from the clutches of the unconscious, and bring in wellbeing through moral and agentive action. Such a view has also influenced the currently prevalent (at times pejoratively used) 'folk psychology' which maintains the possibility for a better understanding of the psychological capabilities we possess and employ in our everyday lives.

A major contender for explaining consciousness using more sophisticated notions about the self, such as representation, in the recent times has been the cognitive sciences supported by neuroscience. Cognitive sciences in general use representational theories to explain the relation between the first person and the second person. Representational theories such as theory of mind when on one hand is successful in explaining how minds deal with the idea of the 'other' in our minds, on the other remove the humanistic and lived content in the conceptualization of the experience. Essentially, embodied experiences are converted into disembodied and abstract contents that require symbols, rules of language and other such concepts for their explanation.

3.3.1 Is Experiential Primacy the Puzzle of Consciousness?

A distinct trend in contemporary discussions on the classic mind-body dualism and the possibility of a unitary self-consciousness started with the theory of the 'easy problems and hard problem' proposed by David Chalmers (1995) which for the first time in the Western world (see Foot note 1, Chap. 2) made a semantic distinction between 'being conscious' and 'what is responsible for consciousness'. Both experimental and cognitive sciences recognized the strong presence of an 'explanatory gap' (Jackendoff 1987) and the need to localize the unity (if any) of consciousness. While Chalmers and a score of other authors who followed him focus on epistemological structures to unravel the puzzle of consciousness, a large number of medical practitioners, therapists and philosophers hail the importance of personal goodness and wellbeing inspired by the wisdom of the Upanishads, Socrates, Kant and Martin Seligman. There is a curious connection between the brain and the mind, individual goodness, and health. Ways of living determine and chart paths to understanding consciousness. Both action and experience count. Describing brain a puzzle, Richard Restak, a neurologist wrote in 1985:

> The brain is the center of conscious experience. It governs the way we perceive, think about, and react to the world; holds our memories in trust; sows, germinates, tends and harvests our emotions; and sustains our sense of self. Granted all that how does the organ work? (Restak 1985, p. 91).

The views which are currently discussed and debated no more fall into a strict division of reductionist and organic approaches. This could be because of the recognition of a distinct characteristic of 'consciousness', that is, the qualitative nature of experience which bridges the first-person and third-person worlds. A prominent view of mutual non-reducibility is that there is a distinction between subjective conscious experience and the biological mechanisms. The argument for such a position is that the first-person data cannot be fully understood in terms of the third-person data. Biological explanations have factored a hierarchy of functions in order to explain consciousness. One such view holds that consciousness is a highly complex motor response occupying 'the uppermost echelon of a hierarchy having the primitive reflex at its base' and that which 'arises from the systems' interactions with the environment' (Cotterill 2001). Another view endorses the 'neuronal group selection' and states:

> ... the brain is a selectional system and not an instructional system like a computer. During the development and behavior of an organism, vast numbers of variant neuronal circuits are generated. These constitute complex repertoires from which circuits shaped by the constraints of value systems are selected to assure adaptive behavior of the organism (Seth et al. 2006, p. 10799).

Approaches to explain consciousness as epiphenomenal, but not in the classical sense of an emergent entity from a physical composite, also take into account the theoretical divide between the empirical and the subjective aspects of consciousness as the primary problem for explanation. Therefore, some of these approaches hold that consciousness 'is formed in the dynamic interrelation of self and other, and therefore is inherently intersubjective' (Thompson 2001) or that it is a system of interactions between the animal and its environment and that it is not located in the brain (Varela et al. 1991). Explanations which address the psychological and social dimensions of consciousness hold that consciousness is 'some pattern of activity in neurons' (Churchland and Sejnowski 1997) or that it is best understood in terms of varying degrees of 'intentionality' (Dennett 1991), and in terms of 'memes' which are the units of cultural evolution (Dawkins 1976; Blackmore 1999). Dennett and Dawkins perceive consciousness as a cultural construct.

Identity theories that equate physical objects and personal attributes that belong to two systems disregard independent existence of the phenomenal quality of experience. Mind is brain, and mental processes are neural processes. Identity theories, especially those which argue for the independent non-existence of experience and mental properties other than in the neural states, are blurred by logical and commonsensical absurdities. Three questions clarify the conceptual and experiential impossibility of physical-experiential identity: if both are one, then why a separate event of an 'experience'?; if the content of experience is identical with a brain state, why does it exist outside the brain?; if experience itself is identical with the neural state, why phenomenal attributes which are sensed and felt in lieu of electrochemical processes?

The primary difficulty with brain-mind identity theories is that the physical objects that are sensed and mental feelings that are experienced are both clubbed under one (physical) category. Obviously, rules that govern color, sound and smell, and those that govern pain, pleasure, anger, joy etc. cannot be the same. Further trouble arises, when it is assumed that experience can be split and deconstructed into the physical sense-data, and the phenomenal content. But, if so a disembodied brain will have sensations and feelings, which is not the case.

All our experiences come as a gestalt. If we see parts to it, it is only because of the objective exercise of cognitive analysis and interpersonal relations that follows. Experience is not constructed from a given set of parts, but is by nature wholesome and immediate and is presented to us in that way.

Another school of thought believes that there are unique neuronal correlates for seeing a red patch, another patch for seeing one's grand-mother, and a third for feeling hungry and that perturbing those correlates will alter its associated percept, or causes it to disappear (Koch and Greenfield 2007). Retaining the possibility of neural correlates, few philosophers and neuroscientists are interested in tracing the subjective components of consciousness represented through the brain in the scientific exploration of meditation techniques (Newberg et al. 2001). This school acknowledges the contribution of Eastern philosophy and wisdom traditions of meditational techniques toward understanding transcendental and extra-ordinary states of consciousness and experiences (Varela and Shear 1999a, b).

3.4 The Harder Problem

In 1984, Kathleen Wilkes in a paper in *The British Journal for the Philosophy of Science* questioned even the importance of considering 'consciousness' as a serious entity for neurosciences:

> … I shall question the existence of a 'problem of consciousness', suggesting that in fact consciousness as such is not at all important, and that psychology and the neurosciences would lose nothing, and gain much, by refusing to chase this will-o'-the-wisp (Wilkes 1984, p. 223).

We are close to three decades after such a conviction was expressed. Are the sciences anywhere near eliminating or disregarding consciousness? Is consciousness still the 'will-o'-the-wisp' that is being chased with no success?

In fact, today neuroscience has embraced 'consciousness' more than ever. Brain sciences have in the past few decades witnessed tremendous progress and impetus in the scientific investigation of consciousness. Brain research and brain scanning technologies revolutionized, along with the growing interest in quantum mechanics and neurophysics, our understanding of consciousness. Therapies and technologies coming together have led to the discovery of causes for several illnesses that have a bearing upon mental functions and self-identity. Alongside the life sciences, cognitive sciences with advancements in artificial intelligence and robotics offered theories that are acceptable to science as well as philosophy.

The central concern of 'scientific approaches' to consciousness is to understand the physiology and neuroscience behind an experience. But then is the first-person completely left out? For reasons not known science finds it difficult to leave away the subjective and first person nature of consciousness. At the same time with no qualms the emphasis given is for a completely reductionistic goal of explaining the non-physical with the help of physical. For instance, Seth et al. say:

> Any scientific study of consciousness is based on the premise that phenomenal experience is entailed by neuronal activity in the brain. Given this premise, an adequate theory of consciousness must be consistent with physics and with evolutionary principles. Nonphysical or dualistic forces or processes must be excluded, and neural mechanisms of consciousness must emerge ontogenetically and provide adaptive advantage to a species via the ongoing exchange of signals among brains, bodies, and environments. Ideally, a theory of consciousness should propose neural mechanisms that account for its various features, which range from the multimodal characteristics of conscious scenes to the emergence of a first-person perspective (Seth et al. 2006).

Primarily, many functions of consciousness are traced to psychosomatic representations that are mapped in the neural system. Since the discussion is centred on the very nature of 'personhood', self and body, have gained the attention of neuroscience as well as social anthropology. Even in a metaphysical discussion on consciousness what gains focus are those processes and concepts which explain the binding of experiences, and the transformation of discrete, quantitative, neural processes to unitary, qualitative subjective experiences.

Yet subjectivity persists to be 'the epistemic object and practical problem' (Langlitz 2010) for disciplines such as neuropsychopharmacology. Such a consideration implies that either what the sciences have conceived of objectivity is limited, or the idea of binding itself to give rise to the subjective is incomplete.

Confronting the 'binding problem' there are two 'astonishing hypotheses'. Francis Crick in his book *The Astonishing Hypothesis* (1995) expounds an epiphenomenal approach which starts with one aspect of consciousness (the visual) to try and find out how it functions, using experimental procedures. Crick speculates that by the end of this century consciousness will be reduced to its neural correlate. In *Shadows of the Mind*, Penrose (1994) draws a triangle of three worlds (which he holds as cyclic rather than linear and hence different from the Popperian 'worlds') such as the physical world rooted in mathematics, mental world rooted in physical structures, and a third world of Platonic truths. Penrose does not believe that consciousness can be founded on physical reality. He with (Hameroff and Penrose 1996) proposes that consciousness arise from processes of quantum coherence taking place in the microtubules (protein structures) in neurons. In order to develop a science of consciousness, according to Penrose, we have to understand how frontier physics and the Platonic world are related.

Functional and operational descriptions of material systems are not readily translatable into properties. It is known that different complex systems manifest utterly different behaviour. There cannot be one to one simulation of properties and behaviours of two systems at various levels. Both functionalist and eliminativist theories disregard a non-natural existence of consciousness. From an experiential perspective there is no explanatory gap since conscious states can be reduced to their causes or to cultural anthropology. Physicalists like Patricia and Paul Churchland suggest that the explanatory gap becomes irrelevant given sufficient amount of neurological detail (Wilson and Keil 2001, p. 304). But such a gap will be filled in when 'folk psychology' gets into the area of neuroscience with advancements in technologies and theories. A strong critic of physical reductionism, Colin McGinn (1997) believes, like Kant who theorized that we can never know the nature of the true world with introspective consciousness, that one cannot know the link between physical brain processes and conscious states. Introspective consciousness cannot provide immediate knowledge of neural states. Neuroscience can neither give access to knowing the nature of consciousness.

It is agreed upon by many that we see what we 'choose' to see. Manifest properties depend upon the observables we choose to look at. Another problem making the puzzle harder is to account for the reversibility of physical processes and conscious experiences, as Chalmers (1995) himself suggests. If a physical process can *lead* to a conscious experience then can a conscious experience simulate corresponding physical structures? This brings us back to the ancient riddle of the egg and the chicken. Does conscious experience come first ordo neural processes appear earlier? It is quite unlikely that any one side will win in this 'who is the first' game. The very nature of a complex entity, if at all we conceive consciousness to be complex like certain physical systems, is that a clean and clear reversal of existence is not possible. The complex interactions, however much are amenable to neuroscience, and their quantitative plottings are not going to give equivalent measures of the qualitative nature of consciousness. The subject and the subjective are just immeasurable.

3.4.1 The Elusive Explanatory Gap

David Chalmers aptly introduces his theory of 'hard' and 'easy problems' with a caveat that 'there is nothing we know about more directly than consciousness, but it is extraordinarily hard to reconcile it with everything else we know' (Chalmers 1999, p. 287). According to Chalmers, the study of consciousness has to distinguish between the 'easy problems' and 'hard problem' and it is with the 'hard problem' that the central mystery lies (Chalmers 1995). 'Easy problems' can come well under the domain of cognitive psychology and neurosciences since they involve the correlating of neuronal mechanisms or physical processes and cognitive functions. We can even expect, says Chalmers, to know how the brain integrates information from different sources and use this information to control behaviour. But the 'hard problem' is hard since we are nowhere near the answer for how physical processes in the brain give rise to subjective experiences. Chalmers defends this distinction with the help of a thought experiment, devised by Frank Jackson, of an expert neuroscientist knowing nearly everything about colour vision but herself colour blind.

Chalmers' position on the exclusivity of qualia brings to focus a contention by the philosopher Nagel (1974) that the material explanation of brain states could never explain the actual inner experience. It is impossible to know 'what it is like to be' someone else, or to have perspective from another's person's or being's point of view. The gap between the science of consciousness and the actual experience can never be filled since we do not have theories and concepts to address consciousness which is a natural phenomenon.

Following Nagel, Chalmers places the 'hard problem' within 'the puzzle of conscious experience'. If we agree that the problem of consciousness is basically the problem of 'I' having a continuous experience in spite of 'my' knowledge or ignorance about the causal connections, then the puzzle becomes that of the conscious experiencer rather than that of the experience. If Chalmers (1995) takes the stand that 'subjective experience seems to emerge from a physical process' (p. 81) and does not deny that 'consciousness arises from the brain' (p. 81), then the puzzle about consciousness will get absorbed by the 'easy problems' without having to isolate the 'hard problem'.

The 'hard problem' gets harder when it comes to the nature of the experiencer who owns the conscious experience. For this reason, the question, 'who is having a conscious experience?' is crucial and perhaps more important than 'what is it like to have a conscious experience?' The problem gets tougher when the relation between the experience and the experiencer is searched. The experiencer or the layered sense of self that owns an experience is the harder problem. The central problem in understanding consciousness is not 'having conscious experiences' but how the self is adhered in and through the varied experiences.

3.4.2 The 'Hard Problem' and its Inadequacies

Dualism begins with the fundamental stance on the connections between neurobiological processes and conscious states. Philosophically the problem is ontological than causal. I might have the knowledge of the physical processes leading to my interest in photography, but that will not answer why I am interested in photography. As John Searle says, '…you can get a causal reduction of pain to neuron firings but not an ontological reduction. That is, you can give a complete causal account of why we feel pain, but that does not show that pains do not really exist' (Searle 1995, p. 63). But then how inadequate is the reduction? Searle writes:

> How does the brain create ontological subjectivity? We know consciousness happens and we know the brain does it. How does it work? How do we approach this problem scientifically? The standard way is to go through three steps. First, try to find the neurobiological correlate of consciousness. A lot of work has been done on this. There is now even a commonly used abbreviation, NCC, for the neuronal correlate of consciousness. Second, try to test if the correlations are in fact causal. Do the neurobiological states cause consciousness? Third, try to formulate a theory. Why do these processes cause consciousness at all, and why do these specific processes cause these specific conscious states? (Searle 2011, p. 50).

Contemporary debates on the 'hard problem' face two inadequacies. The first inadequacy is in framing up a definition for consciousness. It is debated whether or not we should bring the 'unconscious' and other states also into the gambit of consciousness. According to Searle (1995, p. 63), 'consciousness refers to those states of sentience and awareness that typically begin when we begin from a dreamless sleep and continue until we go to sleep again, or fall into a coma or die or otherwise become "unconscious"'. Searle ignores dream and deep sleep states that are inarguably connected with conscious, waking states. To reduce the purview of consciousness to cognitive functions and behavioural patterns in the waking state gives room for explanatory parsimony and not conceptual comprehensiveness. The limited definition of consciousness in terms of the waking state gives isolated importance to feelings and sensations. This leads to the second inadequacy of not considering the contiguity of the experiencer or the sense of self that is adhered in an experience. In an experience such as 'I see a rose' or 'I feel happy', consciousness is the spotlight by being the 'I' and the unique owner of the experience.

The 'harder problem' is to discuss the unitary I-ness which experiences and owns the phenomenon of pain, pleasure, etc. Pain, pleasure, moods and other psychological phenomena cannot be mere narratives of biological functions. Discrete biological functions gain meaning when they accrue to a unitary, continuing self-sense. The 'harder problem' within the 'hard problem' is why or how different conscious experiences accrue to a seamless self-sense.

The 'harder problem' invites a methodological shift and an 'adequate epistemology' as Harman (1994) puts it. The adequate epistemology has to integrate three worlds (with due acknowledgment to Popper and Penrose):

1. The physical world of processes and mechanisms.
2. The phenomenological world of corresponding cognitive and affective functions and associated behaviours.
3. The ontological world of the inclusive core-self.

Often, our discussions stop with the second level. As a result we discuss the mind and the mental in the garb of consciousness. At some point we will have to greet the idea that knowledge of causal connections is trivial as far as the ontology of consciousness is concerned. Otherwise, in spite of amazing neurobiological developments, as persons, we will stay where we started. Inadequate and parochial problematization of consciousness, without considering its ontological nature, will lead to inadequate conceptualization. Such conceptual frameworks might very well throw light on certain biological and cultural traits. However, to believe that the door will open to show the true nature of consciousness is doubtful. Experience gains meaning only in the context of the experiencer. Consciousness has immediacy in our personal lives because of its subjective nature. The subject-object divide is blurred in our experiences.

3.4.3 Subject and Object

The standard neuroscience position is that once neurobiologists identify the neural correlate of consciousness—the electrochemical events that occur in the brain when one has subjective experiences—then they can be tested to find if the correlation is causal. Perhaps the relation is not even causal but identical. There is no such subjectivity bereft of a bodily feedback mechanism. Conscious sensations have evolved by monitoring our responses to input stimuli, and modifying the sensory pathways accordingly. They function to give us a sense of self. (Humphrey 2006); (Dennett 1991) and others who concur with this line of thinking are essentially interested to remove the primacy of self in conscious experience and thereby make consciousness similar to any other biological function.

According to both Searle and Humphrey, whether it is causal or identity relations the subject of consciousness is pervious to and exhausted by neurobiology. According to Searle, 'understanding consciousness is just a matter of neurobiological research' (2006, p. 51), and finding the unified field though there are several philosophical and conceptual difficulties along the way. Searle considers 'brain an extremely difficult *object* to study'.

Why is brain a difficult 'object' as Searle considers? It is largely because there seems to be an impassable difficulty to understand how an object can give rise to the subject. How does the functioning of the physical object, the brain, give rise to a personal subjective consciousness? How or why does the subject come from the physical object? These questions are not foolproof. Why do we assume that subject comes from the object? Is it possible that the subject itself has fashioned the object to be what it is? What is important and relevant are purpose, intention, and meaning of what we sensate.

Perhaps there are no straitjacketed causal and unidirectional connections between the subject and object. The subject-object divide is conceptually strong but fragile from the angle of an experiential stance. It is not just 'seeing a shade of red without necessarily having the concept shade' (Tye 2003; 2009), but seeing red in a context frilled by memories, likes and dislikes, emotions, hopes and feelings. The context gets significance over the otherwise boring singular sensations. When LeDoux (2002) asserts that all that is, is a 'synaptic self', he also concedes that it is an organic self that is biological, psychological and cultural. What is not clear in LeDoux's position is the route from the 'synaptic self' to the 'organic self'. Perhaps for LeDoux and other like-minded neurobiologists the route is not even important.

On a reductionist perspective about sensation we could say that the self is not just a static placeholder to affirm or dismiss the subjectivity of experience. Considering our lived experiences, self is a dynamic entity that changes on its own, changes other selves, and is changed by other selves. Self does not appear to us as the sum of all sensations, since it is *something more* which is revealed only through the personality and attitudes of the person. And, that 'something more' is what adds richness and uniqueness to experience thus making a great difference to our personal lives. Such a self is unavailable in the animal world and hence cannot be understood however much experiments are done with the animals, as against LeDoux's claim. Self is not a collection of processes that lead to sensations. Self is responsible for the mental content *around* and *in* those sensations. Content cannot be replaced by the process.

Since consciousness is best known through one's being conscious and one's experience, self has a major role in defining the parameters of consciousness. Sankaracharya, the founder of the Eastern philosophical school of non-dualism, Advaita Vedanta, (in circa 8th century AD), maintained a theory of consciousness, which emerges from the tension between two standpoints—the sensory content, and the essential experiencer, in an experience. The cognitive equipment, *antahkarana,* according to Sankaracharya, undergoes modification and is subject to physical laws. His metaphysics of consciousness suggest that pure consciousness is not amenable to experimentation and prediction. He emphasizes that the sensory content of an experience and the ontological primacy of the self-sense are not opposed to each other. They are non-dual.

3.5 Perplexing Challenges for Science

A recent paper on explaining the complex neuronal circuitry of the brain as responsible for varied behaviours cites 'thirteen features of consciousness that require theoretical explanation'. These are:

1. Consciousness is accompanied by irregular low-amplitude, fast (12–70 Hz) electrical brain activity.
2. Consciousness is associated with activity within the thalamocortical complex (the 'dynamic core'), which is modulated by activity in subcortical areas.
3. Consciousness involves distributed cortical activity related to conscious contents.

4. Conscious scenes are unitary.
5. Conscious scenes occur serially; only one conscious scene is experienced at a time.
6. Conscious scenes are metastable and reflect rapidly adaptive discriminations in perception and memory. According to the TNGS, qualia are the discriminations entailed by the underlying neural activity.
7. Conscious scenes comprise a wide multimodal range of contents and involve multimodal sensory binding.
8. Conscious scenes have a focus/fringe structure; focal conscious contents are modulated by attention.
9. Consciousness is subjective and private and is often attributed to an experiencing 'self'.
10. Conscious experience is reportable by humans, verbally and nonverbally.
11. Consciousness accompanies various forms of learning. Even implicit learning initially requires consciousness of stimuli from which regularities are unconsciously developed.
12. Conscious scenes have an allocentric character. They show intentionality yet are shaped by egocentric frameworks.
13. Consciousness is a necessary aspect of decision making and adaptive planning. (Seth et al. 2006, p. 10800).

The earlier stand behind the division of 'easy' and 'hard problem' has a strong experimental basis and an idealistic bent at the same time. The current equalization of easy (neural activity) and hard problems (first-person qualia) gets rid of any non-physical element to theorize consciousness.

Perhaps easy problems can be solved in time with medical advances. Hard problem remains unsolvable even with sophisticated physicalist theories. Thus, today, on one hand tangible neural correlates of consciousness are searched for, and on the other mystical and transcendental dimensions of consciousness are glorified.

> Two radically different families of theory currently compete for acceptance among theorists of human consciousness. The majority of theorists believe that the human brain somehow causes consciousness, but a significant minority holds that how the brain would cause this property is not only currently incomprehensible, but unlikely to become comprehensible despite continuing advances in brain science. Some of these latter theorists hold an alternate view that consciousness may well be one of the fundamentals in nature, and that the extremely complex functional systems of the human brain inform this basic property, giving rise to our specifically human variety thereof (Sullivan 2006, p. 59).

The 'hard problem' gets harder not because of the complexity of consciousness but because of and according to the predefined parameters. To correctly estimate the hardness of the 'hard problem' one has to distinguish, as well as integrate, the experiencer and the sensory content of experience. The task is not to arrive at reduced and localized electrochemical contents of experience but to trace, as far as possible, the roots of the self-sense. Certainly, this is a philosophical feat that involves experiments with capabilities for reflection and introspection.

Discussions on localizing conscious states consider consciousness as a 'scientific' phenomenon with the scope for objective investigation. Yet, the experiential primacy of consciousness persists as the puzzle to be solved across interdisciplinary discussions. Essentially, the puzzle is in theorizing the experiential primacy of consciousness as epistemic, psychological or even metaphysical. This is the 'harder problem'. The 'harder problem' is to find a source, that is neither localized materially and structurally in the brain, to hold the ontological essence of consciousness. Is such an effort in the right direction is a question worth deeper reflection.

What makes brain the most exciting yet mysterious *subject* for investigation is its enabling of personal experiences. It is interestingly perplexing that we can be conscious and yet not know what brings about the phenomenon and the phenomenal quality of consciousness.

Let us ask why this is perplexing.

Human knowledge structures are mostly based on knowing the 'other', about an objective world of information pertaining to the 'other'. An ancient Upanishad says that we are created in a way that we look outward, and all our senses are pointed outward.[2] What is different about consciousness is that by nature consciousness 'looks inward'. It is not like any other sense organ of the body that is directed towards external objects. The object of consciousness is inside and internal. Consciousness through the mediation of the mind and the mental structures enables knowledge of an object, whether it is an external physical object or an internal thought. The way we see the world and experience it is based on three orders of realities: the 'I', 'You' and the 'My-World' (Menon 2002, p. 335).

The extrinsic knowledge formation that the knowledge enterprises and epistemological modes of human knowing have been following faces a hump when it comes to consciousness. We feel comfortable when localized knowledge is available about anything which we experience. It cannot be that we do have an experience and still do not know 'how' or 'why' it is there. The availability of 'consciousness' for our most intimate experiences and yet the inability to understand it in terms of neural information makes us concede that consciousness is a complex phenomenon, and that its complexity needs to be addressed. We understand 'complexity' as an intrinsic characteristic of the 'other', and the object of investigation.

This notion of ours about 'complexity' is to be re-examined. What we distinguish as 'simple' and 'complex' need not be the intrinsic characteristics of the object of investigation, but the epistemic structures we have formed based on the availability of third-person information. Though we might be personally aware of our experiences, their representations in terms of cognitive structures and concepts alienate us from what is otherwise so clear and near to our moment to moment feelings. Consciousness invites challenging discourses because of its connections with the personal subjectivity in each one of us, including the experimentalist and the theorist.

---

[2] Katha upanishad: 2.1.1–2.

References

Barkovich, A. J., Millen, K. J., & Dobyns, W. B. (2009). A developmental and genetic classification for midbrain-hindbrain malformations. *Brain, 132*(12), 3199–3230.

Barrett, L., Henzi, P., & Rendall, D. (2007). April 29). Social brains, simple minds: Does social complexity really require cognitive complexity? *Philosophical Transactions of the Royal Society: Biological Sciences: Social Intelligence: From Brain to Culture, 362*, 561–575.

Blackmore, S. (1999). *The meme machine*. Oxford: Oxford University Press.

Chalmers, D. (1999). *The scientific American book of the brain*. New York: The Lyons Press.

Chalmers, D. (1995). The puzzle of conscious experience. *Scientific American, 273*, 62–68.

Churchland, P. S., & Sejnowski, T. (1997). *The computational brain*. Cambridge: MIT Press.

Cotterill, R. M. (2001). Evolution, cognition and consciousness. *Journal of Consciousness Studies, 8*(2), 3–17.

Crick, F. (1995). *The astonishing hypothesis: The scientific search for the soul*. New York: Simon & Schuster.

Dawkins, R. (1976). *The selfish gene*. Oxford: Oxford University Press.

Dennett, D. (1991). *Consciousness explained*. London: Allen Lane.

Edelman, G. M. (1998). Building a picture of the brain. *Deadelus: The Brain, 127*(2), 37–70.

Eriksson, P. S., Perfilieva, E., Björk-Eriksson, T., Alborn, A.-M., Nordborg, C., Peterson, D. A., et al. (1998). Neurogenesis in the adult human hippocampus. *Nature Medicine 4,* 1313–1317.

Hameroff, S., & Penrose, R. (1996). *Orchestrated Reduction of Quantum Coherence in Brain Microtubules: The 'Orch OR' Model for Consciousness* In S. R. Hameroff, A. w. Kaszniak, & and A. c. Scott (Eds.) Toward a Science of Consciousness—The First Tucson Discussions and Debates, Cambridge: MIT Press, 507–540. http://www.quantumconsciousness.org/penrose-hameroff/orchor.html

Harman, W. (1994). The scientific exploration of consciousness: Towards an adequate epistemology. *Journal of Consciousness Studies, 1*(1), 140.

Humphrey, N. (2006). *Seeing red: A study in consciousness*. Cambridge: The Belknap Press of Harvard University Press.

Jackendoff, R. (1987). *Consciousness and the computational mind*. Cambridge, MA: MIT Press.

Joseph, R. (1990). *Neuropsychology, neuropsychiatry and behavioural neurology*. New York: Plenum Press.

Kandel, E. R., & Squire, L. R. (2000, November 10). Neuroscience: Breaking down scientific barriers to the study of brain and mind. *Science, 290*(5494), 1113–1120.

Koch, C., & Greenfield, S. (2007). How does consciousness happen? *Scientific American, 297*, 50–57.

Langlitz, N. (2010). The persistence of the subjective in neuropsychopharmacology: observations of contemporary hallucinogen research. *History of the Human Sciences, 23*(1), 37–57.

LeDoux, J. (2002). *Synaptic self: How our brains become who we are*. New York: Penguin Books.

McGinn, C. (1997). *The character of mind: An introduction to the philosophy of mind*. Oxford: Oxford University Press.

Menon, S. (2002). Structure of mind and structured mind. *Indian Philosophical Quarterly, 2 & 3*, 335–344.

Metzinger, T. (2009). *The ego tunnel: The science of the mind and the myth of the self*. New York: Basic Books.

Nagel, T. (1974). What is it like to be a bat? *Philosophical Review, 83*, 435–450.

Newberg, A., d'Aquili, E., & Rause, V. (2001). *Why god won't go away*. New York: Ballantine Books.

Patten, S. (1976). Hume's bundles, self-consciousness and kant. *Hume Studies, 2*(2), 59–75.

Penrose, R. (1994). *Shadows of the mind*. Oxford: Oxford University Press.

Ramachandran, V., & Blakeslee, S. (1998). *Phantoms in the brain*. New York: William Morrow.

Restak, R. M. (1985). The human brain: insights and puzzles. *Theory into Practise: Learning and the Brain, 24*(2), 91–94.

Searle, J. R. (2006, November 2). *Minding the brain* (Vol. *LIII*(17), pp. 51–55). New York: The New York Review of Books.
Searle, J. (1995, November 2). *The mystery of consciousness* (p. 63). New York: The New York Review of Books.
Searle, J. (2011, June 9). *The mystery of consciousness continues: A review of Antonio Damsio's 'self comes to mind: Constructing the conscious brain* (pp. 50–52). New York: The New York Review of Books.
Seth, A. K., Izhikevich, E., Reeke, G. N., & Edelman, G. M. (2006). Theories and measures of consciousness: An extended framework. *Proceedings of the National Academy of Sciences of the United States of America, 103*(28), 10799–10804.
Strawson, G. (2009). *Selves: An essay in revisionary metaphysics*. Oxford: Clarendon Press.
Sullivan, P. R. (2006). Are current philosophical theories of consciousness useful to neuroscientists? *Behavior and Philosophy, 34*, 59–70.
Tauber, A. I. (2009). Freud's dreams of reason: The Kantian structure of psychoanalysis. *History of the Human Sciences, 22*(4), 1–29.
Thompson, E. (2001). Empathy and consciousness. *Journal of Consciousness Studies, 8*(5–7), 1–32.
Tye, M. (2003). *Consciousness and persons: Unity and identity*. Cambridge: The MIT Press.
Tye, M. (2009). *Consciousness Revisited: Materialism without Phenomenal Concepts*, MIT Press.
Varela, F. J., & Shear, J. (1999a). First-person methodologies: What, why, how? *Journal of Consciousness Studies, 6*(2–3), 1–14.
Varela, F., & Shear, J. (Eds.). (1999b). *The view from within: First person approaches to consciousness*. England: Imprint Academic.
Varela, F., Thompson, E., & Rosch, E. (1991). *The embodied mind: Cognitive science and human experience*. Cambridge: MA: MIT Press.
Washburn, M. (2012). Rethinking the notion of the ego. *Journal of Consciousness Studies, 19*(3–4), 194–222.
Westen, D. (1992). The cognitive self and the psychoanalytic self: Can we put our selves together? *Psychological Inquiry, 3*(1), 1–13.
Wilkes, K. V. (1984). Is consciousness important? *The British Journal for the Philosophy of Science, 35*(3), 223–243.
Wilson, R. A., & Keil, F. C. (Eds.). (2001). *The mit encyclopedia of the cognitive sciences (Mitecs)*. Massachusetts: MIT.

Chapter 4
The Not-So-Rigid Brain: Philosophical Riddles and Experiential Ironies

I am a brain, Watson.
The rest of me is a mere appendix.
—Arthur Conan Doyle, 'The Adventure of the Mazarin Stone'

Is brain prone to change? Recent studies tell us that the brain has the capacity for structural and functional reorganization so as to adapt to internal and environmental conditions. There is established research on neurogenesis where new neurons form even in an adult brain. The brain has immense possibility for growth, renewal, reorganization and is modifiable by experience. Changes occur in the brain from the early developmental years and continue for the rest of the life. As we age, we use both brain hemispheres for performing tasks that otherwise needed only one hemisphere. The brain tends to check for any weaknesses and optimize its resources for better functioning. The brain is at constant vigil.

Brain synapses change with new experiences. This capacity is called 'synaptic plasticity' or 'neuroplasticity' or 'cortical plasticity' where experience causes change in neural firings that enables formation of new connections between neurons. Neural changes are manifest not only in learning and adaptation, but also as a response to brain damage and cortical injuries. The brain has the capacity to transfer functions to adjacent cortical areas from damaged areas and thus lead to functional recovery of the damaged area. A similar phenomenon is also exhibited in the case of amputation. In order to compensate for the loss of the limb and the motor control of the stump, the cortical regions that are responsible for the motor activity of the limb before amputation invade adjacent cortical areas post-amputation.

The brain also has the capacity to switch areas of neural function when the designated cortical area becomes impaired. Brain creates new connections through learning. Attention and emotional relevance lead the way for new connections and their retention. Significant functional changes occur according to decrease or increase in the amount of synaptic connections. Synapses also influences the time involved in the release of neurotransmitters that bring about the neural firing, through action potentials. Changes in brain connections and the neurochemical nexus influence cognitive skills, emotional valences and mental functioning.

S. Menon, *Brain, Self and Consciousness*, Studies in Neuroscience, Consciousness and Spirituality, DOI: 10.1007/978-81-322-1581-3_4,

In the language of neurology, what we describe as a thought or experience is nothing but electrical and chemical changes that are produced in the brain. Since thoughts produce electrochemical changes in the brain, they can be electronically recorded. With technologies suited to record and manipulate these changes, paralysed and disabled people can move objects with their thoughts with the help of interaction with computerized and brain-activated prosthetic devices designed for particular needs. With the help of brain-machine interfaced prosthetic devices that can pick up electric signals associated with movement from the brain, a relation between the thoughts of the subject and the machine is created that modifies body-perception and movement abilities with the help of altered body-maps in the brain.

Findings on the ability of the brain to reorganize and rewire are only a decade and half old, and have questioned the prevailing view that the brain is a finished product with pre-designated areas for functions. The morphology of the brain is determined by genetic factors but its function can be modified by experiences. The brain changes structurally, dependent upon use, and result in acquiring behavioural skills. One of the earliest studies in this field is the discovery that London taxi drivers have a larger hippocampus, the brain area that is responsible for spatial representations and memory by navigation. This study established that the size of the hippocampus and the duration of time spent as taxi drivers were correlated (Maguire et al. 2000). A recent study showed that the correlation between cortical density increase and the time spent as an academic suggests experience-dependent structural plasticity in mathematicians' brains. Increased grey matter density was found in their left-inferior frontal, bilateral parietal regions and inferior parietal regions, the areas that are involved in arithmetic processing and high-level mathematical thinking, which requires visuospatial imagery (Aydin et al. 2007).

Today it is increasingly accepted that the brain can change according to feedback received from experience and how we train our mind. Changes in the brain are not frozen by adulthood. The more active we are, the more we take learning as a lifelong process, the more connections we will form and higher will be our brain density. Neurodegenerative illnesses such as dementia are believed to be absent in brains that have more neuronal density. Memory and the ability to retrieve information at will are dependent on many parts of the brain working together. Our lives have a bearing on the way the brain decides its functionalities and changes. At the same time, our brains operate using feedback from and feedforward to multiple sources—experiential, electrical and chemical.

4.1 Making Sense of Neural Changes

The brain's evolutionary development has paved way for our thinking capabilities in terms of abstract symbols and representations like language. Our cultural lives and accumulation of experiences have helped us to build and preserve a self-narrative with meaningful experiences. A word remains abstract and representational until we give emotional valence to it.

The plasticity of the brain is accompanied by yet another enigma—that the self is somehow able to make sense of neural changes and create corresponding changes in sensations and personal identity. Self-effort, will power, positive thinking, love, compassion, spiritual quietude, and such qualities are found to enhance brain functioning in the case of patients who face mental and physical challenges. Just as there are neural correlates of consciousness, I would like to suggest that there are self-correlates of consciousness. Self-correlates seem to alter the functions of the neural correlates and neural pathways in curious ways.

In terms of brain function, an experience means firing of a cluster of neurons. Firing involves passage of electrical current away from the cell body down to its axonal length. The passage of electric current also activates transference of neurochemicals which function as messengers for the whole body system. Apart from the pervasive electrochemical information system, the neural cortex is also structurally divided to integrate different kinds of information. Different cortical areas are demarcated for highly specialized functions. In effect, this provides a brain map for locations of various functions. Different brain areas work in unison and harmony.

Though it is supposed that sensory and motor functions are localized brain processes, neuroplasticity tells us that the brain has the ability to transfer, extend and take over functions. The brain compensates for lost functions due to neural deafferentation,[1] by creating new connections in the available cortical region. There are evidences for cross-modal reorganization of the brain cortex. The visual cortex of a blind person, for instance, can develop connections in the auditory cortex, resulting in acute hearing. New connections and networks are also created in the case of new learning, artistic capabilities, mystic and spiritual experiences.

Yet another curious discovery brought to light by V. S. Ramachandran in the recent times, and originally by Weir Mitchell in 1871, is about the brain's constant effort to spread on to unused cortical areas, resulting in the experience of the phantom limb[2] (Ramachandran and Blakeslee 1998).

On Weir Mitchell's discovery, Marianne Simmel writes:

> Weir Mitchell coined the term phantom, limb to describe the amputee's experience of the continued presence of a limb which has been lost. Immediately after amputation, as he awakes from the anesthesia, the patient may not believe that the arm or leg has been removed until he can convince himself by looking under the covers. But even once he knows beyond doubt that the extremity is gone, he typically continues to feel it as if it were still present. In the days-and years-to come, the foot of the amputated leg may itch and, as the patient reaches down to scratch it, he reaches for an empty space. He may feel the bed sheets on the arm or leg, he may feel a mild, perhaps pleasant tingling—a phenomenon which Henderson and Smyth regard as basic—or, much more rarely, he may feel pain. He may feel that he can wiggle his finger or toes, flex or extend the wrist or ankle, and that he can perform these movements more or less at will. Despite his knowledge that the amputation has been per- formed the patient may 'forget' and reach out with

[1] Deafferentation is the loss of sensory input from a part of the body caused by injury to (or loss of) the sensory nerve fibres.

[2] The *phantom limb* is an arm or leg that stays in the minds of patients for an indefinite time after it has been surgically removed or lost in an accident. The phantom limb is stimulated by the brain and does not correspond to an actual one.

> the missing hand to grasp something, or to steady himself, or he may step on the phantom foot and fall. At least initially a good many amputees report that they are more aware of the phantom extremity-even though painless-than of the contralateral intact limb, an observation already recorded by Weir Mitchell (Simmel 1958, p. 492).

Ramachandran and Blakeslee (1998) found that in patients who have lost a limb, the area of the brain cortex that processes inputs from the face takes over the area originally responsible for receiving inputs from the now missing hand. He found that in cases of damage to the primary somatosensory cortex, the secondary somatosensory cortex gets reorganized. The brain does a remapping.

The regenerative nature of the brain has made it the 'smart organ', having inherent intelligence to preserve optimal functioning with the help of available tissue and new connections. The final goal in the 'openness' of the brain is to make abstract information and representations meaningful and self-relevant. Association with meaning and self-relevance in turn makes the connections acute and long-lasting. The brain is an organ with flexibility and openness. This most significant characteristic of the brain makes it possible for it to rewire and redefine concepts.

Contrary to the traditional deterministic theory, current extensive research performed by scientists worldwide proves that depending upon the interaction between the person and environment, and responses to the challenges that ensue, the brain develops, learns and grows. Studies in the past decade and half (Schwartz and Begley 2002; Ayedin et al. 2007) tell us that the brain remodels itself throughout life. The brain is capable of forming new neural networks in favour of new learning. It is organized along functional rather than anatomical lines. Different parts of the brain contribute to a single function of the brain.

The brain reorganizes itself by forming new neural connections. The functions of the intact neurons are tweaked and adjusted according to the needs and attention received. In the case of reconnecting to damaged cortical areas, axons of intact neurons connect with the damaged area through new nerve endings, and if one hemisphere of the brain is damaged some of its functions are taken over by the other hemisphere. As we learn we change the structure of the brain. Each time we learn a word a reconnection is made between nerve cells. As we acquire knowledge a rewiring is made in the brain. The intelligent flexible nature of the brain enables it to transfer functions to different areas if a specific cortical area dysfunctions due to stroke. Brain research has documented several cases where the brain increases activity in another region to overcome the loss in one region. The left side of the brain of a right-handed person specializes in enabling music, poetry and mathematics. After hemispherectomy, these capabilities travel from the left to the right side of the brain. In the case of epileptic patients who underwent hemispherectomy, the functions of the absent side of the brain were found to be taken over by the side that was present.

A new area called 'contemplative neurosciences' has emerged in recent times which studies the brain processes underlying contemplative practices such as meditation (Lutz et al. 2004; d'Aquili and Newberg 1993; Newberg 2001), and suggests that the left pre-frontal cortex exhibits pronounced gamma activity during meditation and can cause short-term and long-term neural changes. While patients with obsessive compulsive disorder (OCD) could improve their state of mind through attentive learning and cognitive therapy, the effects of meditation on the brain, according to the studies in contemplative sciences, are far higher. Rick Hanson, a researcher on meditation outlines five steps of attention and suggestive thoughts of wellbeing and positive emotions, as the procedure for a simple practice of meditation.[3]

Hanson suggests that there are enduring positive changes in the brain of those who meditate regularly (Hanson 2011). Those who routinely meditate build synapses, synaptic networks and layers of capillaries which are thicker in the pre-frontal cortex and the insula. The pre-frontal cortex is responsible for the executive control of paying attention and is the seat of positive emotions. The insula is responsible for tracking both the inner state of the body and the feelings of other people, the optimal 'me and the other' divide. The insula is located deep within the brain in a deep fold of the cortex, between the temporal lobe and the inferior parietal cortex. It is made up of two parts and is on the left and right sides of the brain. It is responsible for multiple functions, particularly the mediation of emotions, preparing the body for actions, regulating temperature, and essentially integrating the body with the mind. The thicker insula indicates the potential for increased empathy and better self-awareness. The brain can change according to the thoughts it is directed to, which Hanson calls the 'fundamental skilfulness of self-directed neuroplasticity'.

Today, it is also believed that the development of the brain is not linear. The theory that capacity of the brain to learn increases as an infant matures into adulthood and thereafter diminishes is challenged by the current research findings. The non-linear nature of brain's development is being discussed with enthusiasm. The brain is not 'hard-wired' but its circuits can change and reorganize. The acquisition of knowledge and skills does not happen in linear time but at optimal times. The brain continues to form new neural networks until death if there are optimal environmental conditions and appropriate training. Alongside, studies also reveal that the brain degenerates if it is not used. If other cells do not appropriately stimulate a cell, it self-destructs. The plastic nature of the brain follows the rule of 'use-it-or-lose-it' like in other body muscles. Increase in the use of the specific cortical area results in larger growth or more connections. For instance, it has been shown that the left-inferior parietal cortex is larger in the brains of bilinguals than in that of monolinguals.

There is also a bleak side to the picture of the adaptive nature of the brain. Neuroscience talks about what is termed as 'negative plasticity' where mental illnesses such as depression and anxiety can cause damage to the brain due to neuro-chemical disorders. There is evidence for the possibility that depression can cause

---

[3] The theory and practice of meditation based on Patanjali's *Yogasutra*s suggest various techniques meant for beginners as well as advanced persons for restraining the mind, including the practice of being cheerful. For further discussion, see Chap. 9.

structural changes in the limbic system which is the seat of emotions and memory. The relation between brain structures and emotions are particularly crucial and holistic in the case of mental illnesses. Experience affects brain areas. Brain areas (owing to genetic makeup or behavioural conditions) cause chemical disorders that in turn cause behavioural disturbances.

4.2 The Malleable Brain, 'Me and the Other' Divide, and a Theory of Mind

We do not only experience. We also reflect. We reflect upon our behaviours, intentions, desires, purposes and values. In the process we also imagine what others think, what causes their behaviour, and what their beliefs and value systems are. With a restricted framework for beliefs and intentions, cognitive neuroscience calls such an ability the 'theory of mind'. The malleable nature of the brain is understood when we examine its capacity to also represent the 'me and the other' divide that is fundamentally engraved in our lives. The brain represents events and objects in the form of maps distributed over its parts. 'Theory of mind' is a scientific extension of the experiential base we possess and carry with us all through our lives. Though the 'theory of mind' is criticized for not adequately representing the lived and embodied natures of experiences, it is widely used to understand the inter-subjective nature of the operations of the human mind.

The 'theory of mind' is an agent's capability of representing another individual's mental states, so as to be able to understand, predict and explain their behaviour (Premack 1978). It is suggested that the development of a theory of mind happens in two stages. During the first stage, infants are able to reason with perception and emotion (Tomasello and Rakoczy 2003). During the second stage, when infants are three or four years of age, the fruition of theory of mind occurs and they are able to represent others' beliefs, and respond accordingly. The ability to represent others' minds is found to be present at birth, or immediately after birth (Bosco 1998), and builds on the child's innate ability to share mental states with partners in interaction, and the recognition of agency. It builds on the maturation of the ability to differentiate between those mental states, which are shared and those which are private, as well as on other acquisitions like language and culture (Tirassa et al. 2006).

There are clinical evidences that certain brain impairments grossly violate our otherwise intuitive sense of the 'me and the other' divide, and thus impede social interactions. People who exhibit extreme forms of personality disorder could be substantially impaired with regard to their insight regarding views about others (Oltmanns et al. 2005). People with personality disorders often make their own interpersonal problems worse because they are rigid and inflexible, unable to adapt to the social challenges that they face (Chen et al. 2004).

The 'me and the other' divide has several intricate implications for the malleable brain, and how the brain has to work with the self to change and accommodate personal preferences over a period of life events. As we age, as we cultivate newer values and perspectives, our 'me and the other' divide also changes. The change can be in terms of either thinning down or the widening of the divide. As we include more in our 'me-space' the divide becomes thinner and as we include more in 'other-space' the divide becomes larger. What happens to the brain concurrently is a topic for future investigations. But what we now know is that there are several emotional and physiological attributes that are dependent on the basic experiential divide of the 'me and the other'. Some of these attributes impinge upon our capacities for decision-making, evaluating situations and persons, foreseeing consequences, expressing fear and anxiety, and even having the ability to empathize.

Neurocognitive approaches on a 'theory of mind' have mostly relied on the mental representation of oneself and others, and the inferences people make about each other and themselves. Panksepp says:

> … the cortex generates a detailed map of the world that seems to be re-presentational in some sense of the word. No one has a real good sense of what exactly that means, but people are struggling with it and making substantial progress, especially in areas such as visual and auditory processing. With regard to the all-important subcortical functions that are essential for consciousness—the attentional, emotional and motivational systems—I don't think they are computational in any traditional sense. I don't think you can compute the feeling of hunger (Gallagher and Panksepp 2008, p. 101).

What perhaps will extend the discussion on a theory of mind, that is mostly limited to computationalism and representation of oneself and another person, is an approach that will consider larger experiential categories of 'me and the other' which will include not only people, but also events, relations, values, purposes and other higher capabilities and expressions we possess. Such an approach will help us better comprehend the interrelations between the brain and the self, and their cross-wirings. Meta-cognition presupposes our constant pursuit to include and exclude not just people, but the many interpersonal and intrapersonal attributes that are interspersed in social interactions, and to also personally grow.

4.3 Self-Reflection and Modelling Another Self

The fascinating feature of consciousness is that it is accompanied by a self, rudimentary or full-fledged. When we desire something, or know an object, the intentionality of consciousness is invoked. The fulfilment (or non-fulfilment) of the desire and the knowledge of the object is accompanied by a qualitative aspect of personal fulfilment or personal gain. All our experiences are accompanied by personal feelings towards them, what is technically called the phenomenality of consciousness. The third aspect that closely connects the self to consciousness is the possibility to introspect, be self-aware, and self-reflect in multiple levels.

The significance of the self lies in the fact that it brings in consciousness in a unified matter. Knowledge is always tied to a knower. Experience is always tied to a person. Reflective awareness is always tied to one who reflects. Theories that favour a no-self position argues for the dissociate existence of the experience and the experiencer. For instance, one of the arguments on the dissociative nature of consciousness is:

> When philosophers and psychologists think about consciousness, they generally focus on one or more of three features: phenomenality, intentionality, and introspectibility. I argue that, rather than being three features of a single, noncomposite state, these three features characterize different states of human beings. While these three features can, and often do, occur together, compositely, in human experience, each of the first two can exist independently of each other and of introspectibility. Because of their frequent co-occurrence, the three are taken to be features of a single, noncomposite state (Nelkin 1993, p. 419).

The non-divisive relation between the experiencer and the experience demonstrates that consciousness is unitary. Let us discuss this contention further with the help of our capability to self-reflect. Self-reflection involves awareness about one's mental states and a collective awareness of the personal identity that continues frilled by memories, beliefs, and world views. Reflecting upon another's mind entails complex processes that are facilitated by prior self-awareness. When I think about another person in agony, their existential state (mental, coupled with physical cues) is presented to my self-awareness, which in turn coillumine the general attributes of agony, followed by a comparison and evaluation. In all experiences there is an 'awareness of something' and 'awareness by itself'.

What exactly is 'self-awareness'? It is awareness directed from a first-person to something other than me. The 'other' that is awared is either the (1) the 'other' or the world outside, such as other states of mind, objects, etc., (2) the world inside, such as 'my emotions', 'my perceptions', 'my body', 'my beliefs, 'my identity', etc. Both the worlds require the intervention of self-reflection and participation.

Is there an 'awareness by itself' undaunted by the divide of the 'me and the other'? I wish to speculate that such an awareness resides as the core and can be understood as (1) that binder which unites discrete thoughts, and the two worlds (inside and outside), (2) as meta-awareness of the two awareness' of the inner and outer worlds, and, (3) as the unideated and undivided pure I-ness. Rosenthal calls such a binder as a 'higher-order-thought'. He writes:

> The unity of consciousness is the unity of an individual's conscious mental states. So understanding our sense of such unity requires knowing what it is for a mental state to be a conscious state. I've argued in a number of places that a state's being conscious consists in its being accompanied by what I've called a *higher-order thought* (HOT)—a thought to the effect that one is in the state in question.
>
> … We experience each conscious sensation in relation to every other, as being to the right or the left or above or below each of the others. And, by calibrating such apparent locations across modalities, so that sights and sounds, for example, are coordinated in respect of place, we yoke the sensory fields of the various modalities together into what seems to us to be a single, modality-neutral field. Qualitative states are related in this way even when they are not conscious. But when we are conscious of the relevant mental qualities as being spatially related, this also contributes to our sense of having a unified consciousness (Rosenthal 2003, pp. 325; 329).

Such a *higher-order thought* enables a continuous sense of unity to experience. In Rosenthal's argument:

> Having a conscious sense of unity does not require having an explicit, conscious thought that all occurrences of the mental analogue of 'I' refer to a single thing. We typically have a sense that we are talking about one and the same individual when we use different tokens of a proper name even though we seldom have any actual thought to the effect that such co-reference obtains. The same holds for talking or thinking about oneself using different tokens of 'I' or its mental analogue (Rosenthal 2003, p. 335).

4.3.1 What is a Conscious Experience?

Rosenthal describes the bearer of a thought, the 'I' as one who 'identifying oneself consists of saying who it is that one is talking or thinking about when one talks or thinks about oneself, that is, when one has first-person thoughts or makes the first-person remarks that express those thoughts' (Rosenthal 2003, pp. 334–335). What is more sophisticated about the 'talker' and the 'thinker' is that every time an identification takes place through self-awareness, the self presented is not just a collection of serial reminiscences, but a wholesome light illumining the density of experiencer (talker or thinker) all at one time.

Further, there are three distinct 'features' known of a conscious experience. For instance, at every event of physical pain (physical-conscious experience), mental pain (non-physical-conscious experience) or any (conscious) experience there is a 'gestalt' meaning brought out by a union of three units such as:

the experience (pain),
the experiencer (me *in* pain), and,
the I-ness (me *having* pain).

The first two: the 'experience of pain' and the 'me in pain' are ontologically of a transient nature. Just as I can experience pain, I can also have many other distinct experiences. Correspondingly the 'experiencer ' also changes. The third unit that is of a meta-experiential nature ('me *having* such an experience') is changeless, since it accrues to a continuing and abiding 'I-am-ness'. It is this unit that integrates both the distinct conscious experience and the conscious experiencer and presents a meaningful continuity, and therefore belongs to a core region of the self. The I-am-ness or the core-self presides two functions that are ontologically different. An intentional 'outward' movement of consciousness; and an integral 'inward' movement of consciousness.

4.3.2 The Ongoing Commentary of Self-Report

The initial plane of self-reflection is given and natural to us. Because of self-recognition and initial availability of self-reflection, an ongoing commentary of self-report is experienced by us moment to moment, day in and day out, through physical and physiological dispositions, psychological feelings and social relations. Such dispositions and feelings are internally sensed and immediately available to us.

Thinking about the other, a theory of mind, involves complex processes. A barrage of encoded information is received and decoded both neurally and experientially. When I feel that you are a compassionate person, such a feeling is the result of information received and integrated at various levels. These levels involve:

(a) my distinct self-awareness,
(b) sense of my values and emotions,
(c) my belief in compassion, its existence in others, and its generalist attributes,
(d) my previous experience of compassion in me or in another person,
(e) correlations I already have formed to connect an individual's motivations, and actions with generalist attributes of compassion,
(f) physical (facial, gestural, kinaesthetic) cues received visually from the other person,
(g) judgements generated by the physical cues received from the other person and internal cues received from my body and mind, and,
(h) the matching of cognitive, affective, and visual information that gives a third-person report to my awareness that 's/he is compassionate'.

4.3.3 The Nearness of 'the Other'

We do possess a range of experiences: a certain type pertaining to outside objects, and a certain type pertaining to inside objects. When my toe hits a stone, the pain I feel is 'inside', but the stone, which triggered the pain, is an object outside, which has its own distinct physical properties. The experience of pain is nearer to me than the experience of the existence of the stone. Our experiences are always a negotiation between the nearness and farness of 'the other'.

The feeling of pain is nearer to 'me' than (the perception of) the existence of the stone. At the same time the pain as well as the stone are distinguished from 'me' and is also other than 'me'. The stone as well as the pain are both 'felt' as other than 'me'. There is something unknown about the pain as well as the stone.

Is consciousness 'unknown' like the perceived stone and the felt pain? This question focuses on the 'harder problem' of consciousness. The stone (object with physical properties), or the pain (object with mental properties), are experienced as other than 'me'. They receive meaning when related to an experiencer. Consciousness is not totally unknown, since it is possible to know about it through our distinct experiences. What is unknown about consciousness is what brings about the subjective, meaningful continuity of distinct experiences, and where it can be located in the physical brain.

There is a general agreement that it is interestingly perplexing to be conscious and yet not to understand what brings about the experience of consciousness. The perspectives from the first-person of our own uniquely coloured experiences, and from the third-person of colour-deprived objective data are different not only because of the basic approaches involved but also the very outcomes. Varela and Shear (1999a) made a succinct distinction of these approaches and why it is important to be aware of the distinction.

By first-person events we mean the lived experience associated with cognitive and mental events. Sometimes terms such as 'phenomenal consciousness', and even 'qualia', are also used, but it is natural to speak of 'conscious experience' or simply 'experience'. These terms imply here that the process being studied (vision, pain, memory, imagination, etc.) appears as relevant and manifest for a 'self' or 'subject' that can provide an account; they have a 'subjective' side.

In contrast, third-person descriptions concern the descriptive experiences associated with the study of other natural phenomena. Although there are always human agents in science who provide and produce descriptions, the contents of such descriptions (i.e. of biochemical reactions, black holes or synaptic voltages) are not clearly or immediately linked to the human agents who come up with them. Their defining characteristics refer to properties of world events without a direct manifestation in the experiential-mental sphere; they can only be linked to this sphere indirectly (via the actual laboratory life, the modes of scientific communication and so on). Such 'objective' descriptions do have a subjective-social dimension, but this dimension is hidden within the social practices of science. The ostensive, direct reference is to the 'objective', the 'outside', the content of current science that we have today concerning various natural phenomena, such as physics and biology (Varela and Shear 1999a, p. 1).

The first-person experience gets accepted as a natural kind, or normal or non-mystical, only if it is validated by third-person analysis and representation. Our reasoning frameworks do not approve of 'having something' without knowing 'what it is' or 'how it came'. Is such third-person representation and consensus necessary for all human expressions, is the question. Perhaps, we can possess a complex phenomenon, have many applications of it, without having an objective third-person representation of it in terms of causal and local coordinates.

Damasio famously wrote that the 'first-person' perspective is biological in origin, and it definitely marked the sophistication of consciousness.

When core consciousness began, millions of years and many species ago, we were very far from the current sophistication of modern consciousness, very far from the ease with which we can describe, using language, the reasons behind our actions, past or intended. However, when core consciousness began, we were on the right track and we transcended the critical threshold. We were telling ourselves, without using any words, the answer to the question we never asked, that yes, there was an individual perspective to our percepts, and yes, there was an individual ownership of images, and yes, it was all tied to life (Damasio 1998, p. 1882).

4.4 Self-Reflection and Neurons that Mirror

The ability to reflect is a trait that has been celebrated in both ancient Eastern and Western philosophies. One of the Upanishadic verses traces the beginning of desire to 'having reflected'—'seen oneself' (*so kamayata, bahusyamprajayeyeti*).[4] Is the 'other' a product of self-reflection? The moment we see ourselves

[4] Taittiriya Upanishad: 2–6.

as distinct and as mediated by the process of reflection, do we see the other? Or is it the other way, that we see the other and hence also reflect upon ourselves objectively? The objectivity of our subject and the subjectivity that is entwined with the objective other make our daily experiences rich, changeable, and challenging at the same time.

In 1995, Giacomo Rizzolatti of the University of Parma along with Vittorio Gallasse and other colleagues discovered mirror neurons in their study on macaques. They found that the same set of neurons is fired when the macaques watched an action in another monkey, or when they performed the same action (Rizzolatti et al. 1996). The neurons mirrored or represented the (motor) response of the other individual. Later, it was found that the premotor mirror neuron areas, areas active during the execution and observation of an action, earlier thought to be involved only in the perception and comprehension of actions, were involved in understanding the intentions of others (Iacoboni et al. 2005). They play a critical role in higher order cognitive processes such as imitation, theory of mind, language, and empathy, all of which are known to be impaired in individuals with autism spectrum disorders (Oberman et al. 2005).

Are reflecting about oneself and another object, person or relation, two entirely different processes? How much are they dependent on memories and recollection? How does self-reflection and autobiographical memory influence our capacity to think about others' mental states (Dimaggio et al. 2008)? What are the neurocognitive bases of empathy and self-awareness? How do different aspects of self-reflection influence social cognition? There are some responses to these questions.

Empathy is a key human expression that is studied in recent times in correlation with mirror neurons. The structure of empathy is built on the edifice of 'me and the other' and the forces of desire that ensue. Reflecting upon oneself and one's actions, and mirroring others' emotions and actions, imply a conjoint phenomenon. It is also known that if one is able to clearly articulate one's internal states to another person or to oneself, the same clarity will also be available in the articulation of another's mental states. Reflecting upon oneself and mirroring another's mental state commence from the departure point of 'me' from the other.

We think about ourselves. We also think about others' actions and mental states. Reflection is thinking about the way we think and our thoughts. According to neurocognitive studies, reflecting upon oneself and others together constitute our capacity to socially cognize. Reflecting upon oneself is reporting to self about oneself and therefore is primarily a first-person activity. Reflecting upon another person is a third-person reporting for oneself. Clinical reports on schizophrenia and narcissistic personality disorder show that improved self-reflection may result in better social cognition (Vignemonta and Fourneretb 2004).

Once I know about my mind, I also become aware of that space, the unknown mind, which is outside the realm of my awareness. It is necessary for me to first have a mind in order to reflect upon another's thoughts and actions. If I am aware of another individual's mental states, then it is indubitable that I already possess a self of mine over which I reflect. However, this reverse logic is not a valid reason for the existence of one's consciousness.

But to reflect upon my mind and thoughts, it is not necessary (conceptually) that I am aware of another's mental states, though self-reflection—supplemented by awareness of another individual's mental states, actions, intentions, beliefs and motives—will help me contextualize my thoughts and actions and also have a realistic assessment of the interpersonal relation. The more I am able to reflect upon myself and retrieve events from the narratives I have formed of my past experiences, the more likely I will be sensitive to another individual's mental and physical states. More the accuracy in my mirroring the other person's inner state the more accurate will be my assessment of their intention and the action anticipated from them.

4.4.1 Why Do Neurons Mirror?

The recognition of mirror neurons commenced with studies of monkeys. There is currently intense discussion and research on extending the idea of empathy from the non-human to human animals. Empathy and embodiment go hand in hand at least for a few cognitive scientists and philosophers who endorse the idea of distributed social cognition.

> Mirror systems, in particular, show us how, at the most fundamental neuronal level, our understanding of others is a distributed process that requires action in the world. Hopefully, a better understanding of the embodied and distributed nature of social cognition in our fellow primates will enable us to understand them on their own terms. Tying this to work demonstrating the embodied and distributed nature of cognition in humans … and may then enable us to identify true commonalities cross species, rather than anthropocentric chimera (Barrett et al. 2007, p. 571).

We sense not only the inner world privately available to us through social cognition and interaction, but also the inner worlds of others. We receive information from the external world through sensations, bodily states, and many other physical cues such as gestures, tone in speech, etc. We know about our inner world through our moods, physiological, and mental states, physical disposition, and a self-narrative that is readily available to our awareness at any point of time.

We possess and use self-awareness and empathy to bridge the two worlds of 'me and the other'. The integration of these two characteristics also is essential to determine our psychological and social wellbeing. When the two become disconnected or these functions become hampered, we are faced with cognitive dysfunctions and other pathologies. Developmental biology tells us that the brain functions through the maintenance and stability of the two sides that monitor, influence and direct different actions. The right side of the brain that is responsible for visual and holistic thinking, nonverbal communication, self-narratives and autobiographical memory, develops early in the course, followed by the development of the left brain which is responsible for logical reasoning and verbal language. Together, the brain gives a coherent view of the world, our body and mind.

We monitor our emotions, feelings, and moods, from moment to moment and also as a narrative of our personality. We are aware of our ongoing mental states, the tenor of our minds, and also our personhood as a whole. We develop a view about ourselves over a period of time. As we become adept in monitoring our inner states, we also become sensitive to register others' inner states and respond accordingly. We make assessments. We make changes. We make corrections. Our reflective system continuously feeds the brain with inputs for new learning and new adjustments. The brain in turn directs physiological and physicochemical activities accordingly. Our sense of the self and the neural wirings constantly update and are dependent on the interplay between the first-person report of inner states and the third-person report of other minds. Today, many accept the brain as a social organ—an organ that is responsible for our cultural and social expressions, and an organ that learns according to new associations and feedback.

Earlier in this chapter, we discussed our experiences that are embedded in the 'me and the other' divide. To follow the rule of survival of the fittest, or for the sheer joy of preserving one's existence, we are watchful of the other. In our watchfulness, we represent or recreate the actions of the other and thus attempt to assess their intentions and predict outcomes. In a way, we learn by imitating the other, but with the objectivity to distinguish our own intentions and actions from those of others. Mirroring of actions of the other helps us to move into the private world of the other and share what is in common. We look for cues from various sources: visual, verbal, movement, etc., to recreate and simulate the world of the other, and see what the experience will be like. Mirror neurons help us not to fudge, but to neutrally demarcate the 'me' from the 'other'. The only way to establish a relation between the parts of the divide is to clearly distinguish them, use 'my' embodiment to include the other, and then discover the bridge of intersection. Mirror neuron studies are nascent and time alone will tell us if all the mirroring that we do is for good, and whether what we mirror is imagined or is truly out there.

A recent study at the Ohio State University reported that while reading a fictional story, it was found that the readers themselves feel the emotions, thoughts, beliefs and internal responses of one of the characters as if they were their own (Kaufman and Libby 2012). Researchers call this phenomenon 'experience-taking', an unconscious process which is immersive, when the reader becomes one with the other.

The study on 'experience-taking', scores of studies on our ability 'to project' on to other minds, and mirror neuron research, bring to light like never before that our self-awareness looks for the other's minds and tries to learn about it by simulating and representing it. The other seems to be an existential counterpart of the self, and the schism between self and the other is responsible for developing healthy social interactions and a self-image.

4.5 Implicit, Explicit, and Failing Memories

To define memory is a difficult task. Philosophers, psychologists and neurologists still grapple with the one phenomenon that we all own, and whose presence and absence we are aware of in changing degrees at various points of our lives. We remember many things—people, events, colours, sounds, textures, smells, feelings, and several details that might even fail to have a name.

Memories are engrained in such intricate manner that at times perception, touch or smell brings in a barrage of experiential information to us from the past. Often, we consider memories to bring to us past experiences and impressions. Memories also help us connect to new life events, form new experiences, modify and update old records of previous experiences. Memories remind us of our previous records of experiences and help us anticipate the future. The functions of memory span from the routine job of recall to connecting, ushering and placing new experiences in our self-awareness, thus unfolding a seamless inner and outer life. Without memory, we are unable to connect the past to the present and the present to the past. We create meaning and purpose aided by memories.

Each of our experience is encoded in neural networks, and repeated experiences become increasingly part of similar networks. According to current studies (McClelland and Rumelhart 1986; Rissman and Wagner 2012), neural networks of memory are present all over the brain and are not localized. The distributed nature of memory will ensure that in the wake of a brain damage to a particular region, only the component of experience related to that area is lost, and not the whole of the memory. Clusters of neural firings encode our experiences, form part of networks, and are later retrieved through memory at the trigger of a sensation, perception, or feeling. In this way, the brain ensures that the same set of neurons fire during future efforts of retrieval. It becomes difficult to alter the wirings in the course of time. This phenomenon was described by Donald Hebb, a Canadian neuropsychologist, in 1949, through his famous statement that 'neurons that fire together wire together' (see Doidge 2007, p. 375). An association is formed between neurons that fire at the same time, and they are likely to fire together in the future as well.

Today, this ingenuity of the brain is referred to as Hebb's axiom, and this has important implications for learning and therapies such as cognitive behaviour therapy. It is found that in cases of treating obsessive–compulsive disorder, depression, etc. the mind has an influence on the brain, and thoughts can change the way one's brain would respond. Mind-based therapies can alter the way our brain processes information. They can aid to change our behaviours and responses. Mind by practice can cause the physical structure of the brain to change in order to effect positive changes. That our thoughts and new learning can alter neural connections has implications for treating mental illnesses and cultivating traits such as empathy. By inducing 'positive plasticity' through new learning, behaviours, meditation, positive thinking and other forms of cognitive therapy, psychiatrists believe that the functions of the brain can be regulated to control bouts of fear and anxiety (amygdala), enhance capacities for planning (prefrontal cortex), and decision-making (anterior cingulate), in the case of mental disorders. The brain continues to change for good or bad. But the brain is also adaptive and ready to change according to the training it receives.

4.5.1 Are Memories Functionally Different?

Neuropsychology demarcates two types of memory: implicit (procedural) and explicit (declarative). Nurius (1993, p. 264) compares them to 'knowing how' and 'knowing about'. Implicit memories are formed through the myriad forms of information received through sensations, perceptions and impressions we do not consciously reckon. Without intentional effort, the brain forms mental models and keeps records of experiences that we sense effortlessly. With the same absence of effort we are able to retrieve those records. Different experiences are clubbed together and are represented by a single schema of summary. The brain generalizes experiences through implicit memories. It makes associations between schemas and also helps us anticipate and invoke an action at the onset of intention. An example is driving. Every time I get in to drive my car, I do not have to recall the basic lessons of driving; they come to me with ease as I place my hands on the steering wheel. They come to me in a mechanical fashion without my intentional effort to recall. We perform many tasks in our daily lives effortlessly because of implicit memories. Skills and motor actions are stored implicitly and without conscious awareness.

Explicit memory is memory that we retrieve and recall from the past. They are factual and episodic records of past experiences and events. They retrieve facts and also connect them to the self. In the long run, episodic memories help us form a self-narrative, an autobiographical memory, of our past life incidents. Paula Nurius writes:

> This component of long-term memory contains what is referred to as 'semantic memory' (general concepts about oneself, other people, how the world works) as well as 'episodic memory' (memory of events and experiences in one's life). Semantic memory has been likened to a dictionary or encyclopedia. Episodic memory tends to be organized temporally and to include introspective knowledge of our subjective experiences (our thoughts, feelings, and bodily sensations)-thus the analogy to a movie projector within our heads. Episodic memories of unique events draw on general semantic knowledge to translate and infer meaning of the events, and semantic memories develop through the accumulation and abstraction of information obtained from episodic events. Thus, the two types interact constantly and combine to form knowledge structures in memory and, with increasing experience and complexity, organized clusters and networks of information in memory. Thus arises the notion of 'schemata,' or schemas, for the structures that organize and store information, information in the form of memories of actual events and of abstractions that we generate. A schema is a system of registering information and action in an organized form (an indexing or classification system) and a guide for interpreting subsequent information and action (a schematic diagram or map) (Nurius 1993, p. 265).

While implicit memory becomes available to us moment to moment without our awareness, explicit memory requires attention and focus to build them. Over a period of time we make narratives based on explicit memories and connect people and events. Explicit memories facilitate the lifelong unfolding of experiences with reference to a self and it's past. Explicit (episodic or declarative) memory is deeply private and also influences the self-narrative in significant ways. Our day to day experiences and life events do not separate the two kinds of memories and we do not distinguish them in our actions.

> … episodic memory tends to be more private, self-referential, idiosyncratic, and subjective, it is particularly vulnerable to unbeknownst revision and distortion, unlike semantic memory, which is often based on commonly shared information. Clients' reporting of personal histories reflects less recall, in the sense of backing up a video recorder, than a current construction of that history and its meaning. This gives us insight into why individuals who shared the same experience may later have considerably different recollections of it. In memory, our past is not maintained as a historical record but undergoes change-to a greater or lesser extent as we do (Nurius 1993, p. 266).

Implicit and explicit memories are long term memories, formed over a period of time, lasting months and years. They carry information that we may not use all the time.

There is another set of memories that we use only at times and relevant to only a short period of time. They are short lived and unattended beyond a few seconds or minutes. These are called short-term memories and do not carry information beyond the immediate use. They include memories that are connected to information received through the five senses and verbal information that are relevant only to the given time and do not receive long-term attention. Short-term memories become long term through repetition and association with a self-narrative. The pre-frontal cortex of the brain plays a major role in short-term memory, while hippocampus is the seat of long-term memories. The pre-frontal cortex with the help of the visual cortex and the Broca's area holds information visually and as sound that would repeat for short duration until the purpose of the short-term recall is fulfilled. The question whether damage to frontal lobes will impair memory recalls is answered both in affirmative and negative.

> How the frontal lobes relate to memory depends on the process in question, and the brain region being investigated. Damage in many areas of the frontal lobes does not impair the intrinsic workings of episodic memory, such as en coding. At the same time, lesions in other frontal regions do impair some aspects of memory (e.g., encoding). In addition, some frontal areas are involved in strategic processes, such as monitoring, setting thresholds to discriminate information previously learned from information not learned, and imposing subjective order on the fly. These latter regions are not involved in the representational processes of memory (which are likely more posterior in the brain), but are involved in the strategic, control processes (Stuss and Alexander 2005, p. 86).

4.5.2 Failing Memories for Some, Persistent Memories for Others

While the brain continuously learn and update through forming memories and developing a self-narrative, all components of memories are not intact and are prone to loss due to neurodegenerative diseases. It is increasingly believed now that Alzheimer's disease is a cluster of many types of illnesses, each creating different kinds of dementia (memory loss), and personality changes. Why would brain lose information that is precious for the sane existence of the individual, is a question still in the hands of nature's evolution. How memory loss affects our personalities in an irreversible manner is even clearer when we examine those neuropsychiatric diseases that affect the sense of self and ownership of body and actions.

Literature and biographies amount in big number which describes the extraordinary capacities of some people to remember dates, long strings of numbers, words, and images. Not much attention has been given to the phenomenon of having superior memories when compared to failing memories, and amnesia. There are two classic cases reported, among many, who had extraordinary capacities to remember. The first case is of 'S' reported by the Russian neuropsychologist Luria (1968) who tells us the story of a newspaper reporter who had high retentive powers and visual memory, but no ability to comprehend metaphors and poetry. He was synesthetic, and connected the sound of the word with the meaning. His ability to imagine resulted in a myriad of images in his mind, and difficulty in distinguishing reality from what is imagined. Luria writes:

> To me there's no great difference between the things I imagine and what exists in reality. Often, if I imagine something is going to happen, it does. Take the time I began arguing with a friend that the cashier in the store was sure to give me too much change. I imagined it to myself in detail, and she actually did give me too much change of 20 rubles instead of 10. Of course I realize it's just chance, coincidence, but deep down I also think it's because I saw it that way (Luria 1968, p. 146).

Luria's 'S' remembered and imagined lurid details but most of them were unrelated and insignificant. Most of us do not have memory of our experiences before the age of three or four, and our memory declines by age as well. But what if all that one remembered pertained to the minutest autobiographical detail from early childhood? A study published in *Neurocase* reports the unusual story of a woman called 'AJ' who did not use mnemonic strategies like Luria's 'S' but was innately endowed to remember all trivial details of personal experiences from the age of 11 with unprecedented accuracy. The paper quotes from one of the conversations with 'AJ':

> I am thirty-four years old and since I was eleven I have had this unbelievable ability to recall my past, but not just recollections. My first memories are of being a toddler in the crib (circa 1967) however I can take a date, between 1974 and today, and tell you what day it falls on, what I was doing that day and if anything of great importance (i.e.: The Challenger Explosion, Tuesday, January 28, 1986) occurred on that day I can describe that to you as well. I do not look at calendars beforehand and I do not read twenty-four years of my journals either. Whenever I see a date flash on the television (or anywhere else for that matter) I automatically go back to that day and remember where I was, what I was doing, what day it fell on and on and on and on and on. It is non-stop, uncontrollable and totally exhausting (Parker et al. 2006, p. 35).

Parker et al., who studied 'AJ', distinguished her capacity to recollect and retain personal details of her life from the feats possessed by 'S' and others who retained vast amount of information of no personal significance. The phenomenon of extraordinary capability of 'AJ' to remember and retain autobiographical information of her life time since she was a toddler with accurate details was named 'hyperthymestic syndrome' by the researchers.

4.5.3 The Truth Behind Memories

Another debate that is not recent but perhaps commenced from the times of ancient philosophy is the relation between memory and self-recognition. Is self a fiction created by the self-recognition that occurs during memory recall? One of the recent proponents of such a view says:

> What appears to be a loss of memory is in reality an inability to create, rapidly, complex motor coordination. Memory, then, is not a set of stored images that can be remembered by an independent 'I'; memory is a set of ever-evolving procedures. And the brain's abstractions of those procedures, 'three dimensionality,' 'distance,' the idea of 'memory' and so on, must also evolve. Hence our 'identity,' our personality, is the brain's reproduction of the totality of our 'memories' and 'experiences.' And though we have many different ideas about who we are (and of who others are), ultimately there are limits to our own understanding, just as there are limits to the understanding a blind man who has acquired sight can have of his physical surroundings. We recognize ourselves as persons in terms of our relation to others, and at each new encounter we reconstruct our identity, just as we reconstruct the motor acts that make up speech as we listen to others. The brain's abstraction of the reconstruction, the synthesis that is our basis of recognition (and ultimately our understanding) of what we have just heard, is what memory is; and a personality, an identity, is an analogous reconstruction of an 'I' in new situations. Paradoxically we understand the abstraction of memory as somehow separate from our personality and yet a part of it (Rosenfield 1995, p. 202).

An ever exciting philosophical discussion on memory is about the 'truth' behind it. How much of a memory is true to the corresponding original experience? Any time we recall a memory do we reconstruct the event using what is called in cognitive sciences 'traces of memory' and its relevance at that point of time? On one count, we cannot live sanely without memories, and on another count, our memories on recall need not result in the actual representation of an event stored in the brain. Even though the content of memory can have elements of both imagined outcomes or objects, and the actual event that occurred in the past, the act of recall happens in the now of the time. The 'presentness' of the act of recall indicates our innate ability to distinguish between events in the past and their relation to the events in the present. The past and the present are connected through the actual act of recall with the help of a self-narrative which is built along our life experiences and emotional filtering. The sheer fact that we believe in what we recalled as having existed sometime in the past, according to Reid, has to presuppose a self that existed and underwent the contents of the experiences in the past. Reid writes:

> The remembrance of a past event is necessarily accompanied with the conviction of our own existence at the time the event happened. I cannot remember a thing that happened

> a year ago without a conviction as strong as memory can give, that I, the same identical person who now remember that event, did then exist (Reid 1994, p. 208).

Memories are mostly our 'impressions' about past events and not exact photographs of the past experiences. Perhaps the auditory and visual memory, we possess of numbers, objects, and faces, can be recalled as they are, while experiences and associations connected with abstract symbols, words, numbers and objects are prone to expectations and objectivity we possess as unique individuals. Hence, what we recall are not just reproductions of what happened in a past time, but more the reinterpretation of a past experience. Our self-narratives continue to influence the content of the recalled experience and the reinterpretation is guided by the 'me and the other' divide that we continue to update. The divide between 'me and the other' influences our capacities for objective assessment of responses, which result from the interactions with the 'the other'. And once again, objectivity or an accurate representation of reality is possible by the dual process of a clear distinction of the qualities of two parts of the divide, and thereby minimizing 'my' projections, followed by the space of 'me' extending its limits to inhabit the space of 'the other'.

4.6 Brain and the Subjective Markers of Meaning-Making

Are neural pathways traceable in a neat manner for complex experiences such as visual (and other sensory) experience or the ability to be compassionate? Is it possible to accurately trace the neural correlates of compassion and love? How is information from complex and characteristically different sources collated and 'stored' to guide futuristic actions and responses? These questions point to a central concern: the neural and subjective markers of brain's collective intelligence.

Our experiences can modify patterns of neural firings and create new networks according to our needs. The brain-mind-person complex is a lifelong learner from experiences and is open to adaptation and adjustments at many levels. Experiential factors shape the neural circuits underlying social and emotional behaviour from the prenatal period to the end of our lives through incidental influences of the environment and intentional influences through interventions (Davidson and McEwen 2012). Even without our conscious participation there is a two-way communication between our experience and the biology of the brain. The information that we receive from the sensory world, and the inner world of emotions, influence the way we think and make decisions.

In fact, according to current neuroscience, most of our experiences are the result of an optimal exchange between that part of the cortex responsible for reasoning, and abstract representations, with the limbic region responsible for emotions and personal reference. The anterior cingulate cortex (ACC), an area in the middle prefrontal cortex, is the region that focuses our attention and mediates sensations that we receive from the body and feelings from interactions with others. The ACC connects our physical body and mind with the world of 'the other'. It is the limbic system that labels our experiences as pleasing or uncomfortable. It is now known that the middle prefrontal cortex along with the limbic system integrates self-awareness with information received from the external world, and gives us self-relevant and meaningful experiences.

All our perceptions are a combination of the information we receive through our senses and the prior learning and memories we possess. The experience that is finally presented to our self-awareness is not a raw sensation, but that which is weighed by the associations we have made in the past. Each of our experiences is presented after being filtered through our feelings, memories, attitudes, beliefs, value systems and the self-narrative with which we stitch all of these together. Our self-awareness (the awareness of our inner and physical states) coupled with the information received from 'the other', through the models we simulate, functions as the subjective marker in the process of making meaning out of what is presented to us every moment as experience. The not-so-rigid brain gets support when our 'me' sense and 'the other' sense coexist and pervade into each other without losing the defining characteristics of each world.

Is 'me and the other' a fundamental divide that we cannot do away with? Is it the basis of the neural and subjective markers for the collective intelligence of brain? The discussion about consciousness is discussion about experience, and the discussion on experience is about the implicit divide fundamental to its structure. The discussion on experience is a discussion about the 'self'. 'Experience' and 'self' certainly relate to something that is more than what happens in the brain, more than pathological conditions, more than everyday life events, more than transcendental states.

I would suggest that behind and beneath the fundamental psychological and phenomenological divide of 'me and the other' is the existence of a unitary consciousness which some call the 'being' or 'ipseity' or 'amness'. As long as the 'me and the other' divide that makes our psychological space clean and functional is not disruptive, we may not be sensitive to the underlying deeper origin of the divide. But once the divide is affected in pathologies, or even in conflicting challenges presented by life events, the core being, or the core-self, becomes important and serves as the realm from where once again the clarity for the divide and its healthy coexistence is drawn. To consider the biological brain as the primary arbiter for consciousness, and brain itself as the person, will perhaps help empirical sciences, but this is not a viable view for the human sciences. For instance, Gregory Nixon writes:

> Since educators are always looking for ways to improve their practice, and since empirical science is now accepted in our worldview as the final arbiter of truth, it is no surprise they have been lured toward cognitive neuroscience in hopes that discovering how the brain learns will provide a nutshell explanation for student learning in general. I argue that identifying the person with the brain is scientism (not science), that the brain is not the person, and that it is the person who learns. In fact the brain only responds to the learning of embodied experience within the extra-neural network of intersubjective communications. Learning is a dynamic, cultural activity, not a neural program (Nixon 2012, p. 298).

What needs to be taken into consideration is that what we are talking about, the complexity of the human brain, is the result of the combination of our evolutionary and biological base, personal and collective history, and several experiments in culture. The brain itself is an outcome of complex biological and cultural processes, and hence is a work in progress.

4.7 Philosophical Riddles and Experiential Ironies

The questions we ask about consciousness have their bases on different kinds of experience: dream state, waking state, memory, feelings, beliefs, etc. The major epistemological worry faced by the neurologist, the philosopher, and the psychologist, is the commonest expression of the central feature of consciousness, that is, 'experience'.

Alongside the 'experience' is the key to the riddle, that is, 'agency', which is a fascination not just for cognitive scientists and psychologists, but also for social scientists and philosophers. When on one side 'agency' posits the space for experimentation onto understanding the minimal nature of a selfhood, on the other it raises fundamental questions on freewill, choice-making and responsibility. Life sciences and social sciences have to consider the fact that human agency embodies a multitude of objects and processes in its field that we may take for granted in daily life.

> [T]here are many ways in which sub-personal processes are constitutive of human agency and action. These processes involve both physiological and cognitive processes within the body and material realities outside it. Depending on the way we choose to understand the latter (the external, material elements that constitute agency and action), they can be categorized as physico-chemical, ecological, or technological, elements. Therefore, we propose that social scientists also attend to the chemistries, ecologies and technologies that human actions embody. This would improve the understanding of how social interaction and social structures empower, or disempower, agents in affecting the material constituents of their own - the agents' - capacity to perform action (Bruun and Langlais 2003, p. 46).

The notion of agency brings in with ease neurological, neuropsychiatric, social and ethical questions. Are such questions amenable to a reductive neuroscientific purview?

This worry is epistemically described as how to have a theoretical explanation for the mutual influence of neural events and subjective experiences, and which is the defining characteristic of consciousness. Attempts to understand 'experience', whether it is simple, physical pain or a much more complex, psychological pain, will have to cross the epistemological barriers of hierarchies and causal relationships, demanding a non-linear path, if we have to understand its subjective nature and the agent who seems to be the apparent master behind the mystery.

The classical description of consciousness as 'unitary' has evolved—in order to accommodate the questions emerging in interdisciplinary dialogues—to present the term 'self', which was once considered metaphysical, but which is very much available for scientific discussion today. The epistemological transition from a third-person perspective to a first-person perspective will be able to accommodate the ironies and idiosyncrasies that our experiences come with.

There is an interesting and serious turn of route taking place in current discussions on consciousness. This turn is based on and compelled by the intractable relationship of consciousness with 'experience', and the 'me and the other' divide on which experience is embedded. The closest empirical correlate for the unity and subjective nature of consciousness is 'experience'. In any experience the cognitive, affective and sensory aspects are united in a well-integrated manner. But at the same time the content of an experience can be studied based on at least an apparent division of it into sensory, cognitive and affective elements. Hence, the scientific focus on 'experience' in the discussion on consciousness.

What is intriguing is that though there is the recognition of experience as vital in the study of consciousness, the goal of mainstream methodologies is to strip 'experience' off, or to convert human qualities to attributes of artificial systems, or to generalize the functionalities to a common animal world. The qualities characteristic of an experience (unitary and subjective) are made available to such approaches of study on the basis of empirical standards such as causal connections, neural influences, neural locations, social behaviour, etc. But, the interesting commonsensical fact is that such studies do not replace qualities but only give an alternate *lingua franca* for descriptions.

If our research guidelines are not based on our basic premise to study consciousness (experience, which is unitary and subjective), then certainly we cannot make a claim that brain studies apart from giving new knowledge about brain functions will also lead to a complete theory of consciousness. The puzzle in the current discussions on consciousness is that of the persistent conflict between brain sciences and phenomenology, and their joint influence in understanding the ontology of consciousness.

References

Aydin, K., Ucar, A., Oguz, K., Okur, O., Agayev, A., Unal, Z., et al. (2007). Increased gray matter density in the parietal cortex of mathematicians: A voxel-based morphometry study. *American Journal of Neurobiology, 28*, 1859–1864.

Barrett, L., Henzi, P., & Rendall, D. (2007, April 29). Social brains, simple minds: Does social complexity really require cognitive complexity? *Philosophical Transactions of the Royal Society: Biological Sciences: Social Intelligence: From Brain to Culture*, 561–575.

Bosco, F. M. (1998). Sharedness as an innate basis for communication in the infant. *Proceedings of the 20th Annual Conference of the Cognitive Science Society.* Mahwah, NJ: Erlbaum.

Bruun, H., & Langlais, R. (2003). On the embodied nature of action. *Acta Sociologica, 46*(1), 31–49.

Chen, H., Cohen, P., Johnson, J., Kasen, S., Sneed, J., & Crawford, T. (2004). Adolescent personality disorders and conflict with romantic partners during the transition to adulthood. *Journal of Personality Disorders, 18*, 507–525.

Damasio, A. R. (1998). Investigating the biology of consciousness. *Philosophical Transactions: Biological Sciences—The Conscious Brain: Abnormal and Normal, 353*(1377), 1879–1882.

d'Aquili, E., & Newberg, A. (1993). Liminality, trance and unitary states in ritual and meditation. *Studia Liturgica, 23*, 2–34.

Davidson, R., & McEwen, B. (2012). Social influences on neuroplasticity: Stress and interventions to promote well-being. *Nature Neuroscience, 15*, 689–695.

Dimaggio, G., Lysaker, P., Carcione, A., Nicolo, G., & Semerari, A. (2008). Know yourself and you shall know the other…to a certain extent: Multiple paths of influence of self-reflection on mindreading. *Consciousness and Cognition, 17*, 778–789.

Doidge, N. (2007). *The brain that changes itself: Stories of personal triumph from the frontiers of brain science*. Penguin Books.

Gallagher, S., & Panksepp, J. (2008). How to undress the affective mind: An interview with Jaak Panksepp. *Journal of Consciousness Studies, 15*(2), 89–119.

Hanson, R. (2011, April). *Institute of Noetic Sciences*. Retrieved May 10, 2012, from http://www.noetic.org/noetic/issue-nine-april/self-directed-neuroplasticity/.

Iacoboni, M., Molnar-Szakacs, I., Gallese, V., Buccino, G., Mazziotta, J., & Rizzolatti, G. (2005). Grasping the intentions of others with one's own mirror neuron system. *PLoS Biology, 3*(3), 0529–0535.

Kaufman, G. F., & Libby, L. K. (2012). Changing beliefs and behavior through experience-taking. *Journal of Personality and Social Psychology*.

Luria, A. (1968). *The mind of a mnemonist: A little book about a vast memory*. New York: Basic Books.

Lutz, A., Greischar, L. L., Rawlings, N. B., Ricard, M., & Davidson, R. J. (2004). Long-term meditators self-induce high-amplitude gamma synchrony during mental practice. *Proceedings of National Academy of Sciences, 101*(46), 16369–16373.

Maguire, E., Gadian, D., & Johnsrude, I. (2000). Navigation-related structural change in the hippocampi of taxi drivers. *Proceedings of the National Academy of the Sciences of the USA* (pp. 4398–4403).

McClelland, J. L., & Rumelhart, D. E. (1986). Amnesia and distributed memory. In J. L. McClelland & D. E. Rumelhart (Eds.), *Parallel distributed processing: Explorations in the microstructure of cognition* (Vol. 2, pp. 503–527). Cambridge, MA: MIT Press.

Nelkin, N. (1993). What is consciousness? *Philosophy of Science, 60*(3), 419–434.

Newberg, A., d'Aquili, E., & Rause, V. (2001). *Why God won't go away*. New York: Ballantine Books.

Nixon, G. M. (2012). You are not your brain: Against "Teaching to the Brain". In D. King, & K. Dyer (Eds.), *International handbook of academic research and teaching: Proceedings of intellectbase international consortium* (Vol. 22, pp. 298–306). San Antonio.

Nurius, P. S. (1993). Human memory: A basis for better understanding the elusive self-concept. *Social Service Review, 67*(2), 261–278.

Oberman, L. M., Hubbard, E. M., McCleery, J. P., Altschuler, E. L., Ramachandran, V. S., & Pineda, J. A. (2005). EEG evidence for mirror neuron dysfunction in autism spectrum disorders. *Cognitive Brain Research, 24*, 190–198.

Oltmanns, T. F., Gleason, M. E., Klonsky, E. D., & Turkheimer, E. (2005). Meta-perception for pathological personality traits: Do we know when others think that we are difficult? *Consciousness and Cognition, 14*, 739–751.

Parker, E. S., Cahill, L., & Mcgaugh, J. L. (2006). A case of unusual autobiographical remembering. *Neurocase, 12*, 35–49.

Premack, D. (1978). Does the chimpanzee have a theory of mind. *Behavioral and Brain Sciences, 1*, 512–526.

Ramachandran, V. a. (1998). *Phantoms in the brain*. New York: William Morrow.

Ramachandran, V., & Blakeslee, S. (1998). *Phantoms in the brain*. New York: William Morrow.

Reid, T. (1994). In R. E. Beanblossom, & K. Lehrer (Eds.), *Inquiry and essays*. Indianapolis: Hackett.

Rissman, J., & Wagner, A. (2012). Distributed representations in memory: Insights from functional brain imaging. *Annual Review of Psychology, 63*, 101–128.

Rizzolatti, G., Fadiga, L., Gallese, V., & Fogassi, L. (1996). Premotor cortex and the recognition of motor actions. *Cognitive Brain Research, 3*, 131–141.

Rosenfield, I. (1995). Memory and identity. *New Literary History: Narratives of Literature, the Arts, and Memory, 26*(1), 197–203.

Rosenthal, D. M. (2003). Unity of consciousness and the self. *Proceedings of the Aristotelian Society, New Series, 103*, 325–352.

Schwartz, J. M., & Begley, S. (2002). *The mind and the brain: Neuroplasticity and the power of the mental force*. New York: HarperCollins Publishers.

Simmel, M. L. (1958). The conditions of occurrence of phantom limbs. *Proceedings of the American Philosophical Society, 102*(5), 492–500.

Stuss, D. T., & Alexander, M. P. (2005). Does damage to the frontal lobes produce impairment in memory? *Current Directions in Psychological Science, 14*(2), 84–88.

Tirassa, M., Bosco, F. M., & Colle, L. (2006). Rethinking the ontogeny of mindreading. *Consciousness and Cognition*, 197–217.

Tomasello, M., & Rakoczy, H. (2003). What makes human cognition unique. From individual to shared to collective intentionality. *Mind and Language, 8*, 121–147.

Varela, F. J., & Shear, J. (1999a). First-person methodologies: What, why, how? *Journal of Consciousness Studies, 6*(2–3), 1–14.

Vignemonta, F. d, & Fourneretb, P. (2004). The sense of agency: A philosophical and empirical review of the "Who" system. *Consciousness and Cognition, 13*, 1–19.

Chapter 5
Body-Sense and Self-Sense: Why is Minimalism Insufficient?

Consciousness is the appearance of a world
—Metzinger, 2009
World is the appearance of consciousness

—Sankaracharya, circa 8 c. CE

Many of us have read Francis Crick's *The Astonishing Hypothesis*, published in 1995 with the subtitle *The Scientific Search for the Soul*. Though Crick's primary interest was in genetic structures, subsequently he became interested in consciousness. His astonishing hypothesis is that:

> 'You', your joys and your sorrows, your memories and your ambitions, your sense of personal identity and free will, are in fact no more than the behavior of a vast assembly of nerve cells and their associated molecules. As Lewis Carroll's Alice might have phrased it: 'You're nothing but a pack of neurons!' (Crick 1995, p. 3).

Let us give attention to the word 'you' used in quotes by Crick. For Crick, 'you' is a non-entity since it is *no more than* the behaviour of a vast assembly of nerve cells. It is not sufficient to talk about a concept of the self. The subtitle of his book, *The Scientific Search for the Soul*, is a sarcastic expression. There is nothing called soul. And there is nothing for science to look into if at all there is something called 'soul'. Crick is not interested in the concept of 'self' (the usage of which would indicate a non-mystic connotation). For Crick, 'self' is best expressed as 'soul' to indicate its absolute non-existence, and therefore its irrelevance.

Years have passed since Crick published his 'astonishing hypothesis'. It astonished a few. Since then many papers have been written on the self. Today, the idea of the self is one of the most important problems for neuroscience, neuropsychiatry and neuropsychology. It is no more a philosophical muddle for the neurosciences. But it is an important puzzle to be solved, and beckons attention for empirical investigation.

What exactly is the nature of such a puzzle which was dismissed by Crick? The fundamental puzzle is the question, 'Is my inner awareness of my-self separate from my body?' Basically, is my body-sense separate from my self-sense? What are

S. Menon, *Brain, Self and Consciousness*, Studies in Neuroscience, Consciousness and Spirituality, DOI: 10.1007/978-81-322-1581-3_5,

body-sense and self-sense? The most prevalent approach is of reductionism—neural or computational—to a basic, primitive, unessential, abstract self, which has cortical origins, or, to an emergent property that can be simulated in an artificial system.

One of the interesting portrayals of self in recent times as illusory is that of Dennett (1991, 1996) who separates the self from the body with certainty, but only to equate it with a narrative fiction, and hence as existing nowhere. If one dissociates all functions and functional distinctions from consciousness, if the puzzle of experience is supposed to be something above and beyond the performance of cognitive and behavioural functions, then, according to Dennett (1996), there is nothing else to wonder about. For Dennett, there is no minimal or embodied self, but only a self that is created in one's own biographical fiction. He says:

> A self, according to my theory, is not any old mathematical point, but an abstraction defined by the myriad of attributions and interpretations (including self-attributions and self-interpretations) that have composed the biography of the living body whose center of narrative gravity it is. As such it plays a singularly important role in the ongoing cognitive economy of that living body, because, of all the things in the environment an active body must make mental models of, none is more crucial than the model the agent has of itself (Dennett 1991, p. 427).

Searle makes an interesting statement criticizing assumptions that support functional reductionism:

> ... all of these reductionist attempts to eliminate consciousness are as hopeless as the dualism they were designed to supplant. In a way they are worse, because they deny the real existence of the conscious states they were supposed to explain. They end up by denying the obvious fact that we all have inner, qualitative, subjective states such as our pains and joys, memories and perceptions, thoughts and feelings, moods, regrets, and hungers (Searle 1997, p. xiii).

According to Jonathan Shear, the subjective self is the hard problem that requires better scientific investigation. He writes:

> ... a well-developed science of the subjective phenomena of consciousness might turn out to transform our understanding of the hard problem incomparably unexpected ways. (Shear 1996, p. 58).

If we concede that there is something called self-sense and that it is separate from the body-sense, further questions are: are these two senses distinct? ; if not, how are they entangled since I experience them together?; and perhaps the most interesting question for all of us is what constitutes these basic everyday senses? How is it possible that we have a neat, clear sense of our body and our self? What is it to sense at all?

5.1 Making Sense of 'Sense'

In day-to-day parlance the word 'sense' implies a meaning intended or conveyed. For example, we might say 'what you say makes sense' to me. Another idea of sense is to be aware, or have clear thinking. For example, we might say, 'finally he came to his senses'. The third possibility of 'sense' is a vague or little awareness, such as 'I get a sense that something is not okay'. Another set of meanings for 'sense' is the faculty to perceive (sight, hearing, smell, taste and touch), the ability to move and assess posture (proprioceptive sense), and, the fundamental and closest feeling of I-am-ness.

Are the self-sense and the body-sense distinct senses? A dominant approach inspired by Aristotelian thinking is that the self-sense *is* the body-sense. Who I am is closely tied to my embodied existence. I cannot sense myself without the accompanying body-sense. Another view, perhaps more of idealist intent, is that self-sense is not just a sense but the *essence*. I-am-ness is essential and the core. Embodiment is only one aspect of the self-sense. Such a view is not new and commenced from the time of the Upanishads in the East and Pythagoras in the West, later developed by Plato, Augustine and Descartes.

The extreme view is to attribute non-existence to the sense of self. The vociferous champion of this view is Thomas Metzinger who equates the sense of self with yet another phenomenal experience, just as smell or taste. He writes:

> What exactly does it mean to have the *conscious experience* of being someone? In this limited sense, the folk-phenomenological notion of 'being someone' denotes a phenomenal property like many others, a property like the scent of mid amber and sandalwood or the gustatory experience of cinnamon, a property like the emotional experience of elation, or the sense of surprise going along with a sudden cognitive insight. It is just a way of experiencing reality: currently, you *are* someone. What makes consciously experienced selfhood special, and different from all the other forms of experiential content, is the fact that—in nonpathological standard situations and in beings like ourselves—it is highly invariant. It is *always* there.
>
> This phenomenally transparent representation of invariance and continuity constitutes the intuitions that underlie many traditional philosophical fallacies concerning the existence of selves as process-independent individual entities, as ontological substances that could in principle exist all by themselves, and as mysteriously unchanging essences that generate a sharp transtemporal identity for persons. But at the end of this investigation we can clearly see how individuality (in terms of simplicity and indivisibility), substantiality (in terms of ontological autonomy), and essentiality (in terms of transtemporal sameness) are not properties of selves at all. At best, they are folk-phenomenological constructs, inadequately described conscious *simulations* of individuality, substantiality, and essentiality. And in *this* sense we truly are no one. We now arrive at a maximally simple metaphysical position with regard to selves: No such things as selves exist in the world (Metzinger 2003, p. 626, italics in original).

An immediately noticeable mistake that Metzinger makes is to include self-sense in the category of percepts and sensory feels. If self-sense is another feel, then how and why does this grand-feel persist and continues to hold and showcase all other feels, is a valid question. Moreover, though it is empirically easier to conceptualize embodiment and the self-sense as one, experientially it is otherwise. To understand our identity with body parts and body as a whole, to recognize the illusoriness and reality of that body (or parts) which we own as ours, to relate to the representation of the body and its changing contours, require the distinction between the body-sense, the self-sense and the inclusive core-self.

5.2 What is Body-Sense?

Body-sense is primarily a combination of internal senses such as pain, balance, thirst and hunger. We experience different kinds of pain, ranging from a pin prick to much intense toothaches. We are able to walk without conscious thought of the body-sense and without the constant fear of falling, because of the balance that accompanies without our conscious thought. Our living is also marked by the two inner senses of thirst and hunger. These aside, we have the external senses for hearing, vision, taste, touch and smell. We exteroceptively and interoceptively relate with the world through the panoply of senses and the body-mind complex.

5.2.1 Brain Cartography and the Body-Sense

According to the theory of brain maps, every point of our body is plotted and systematically represented in the brain to form body maps. In the brain, distributed in the occipital, parietal, frontal and temporal lobes, there are patches of tissues dedicated to represent each of our body parts. The brain forms mini-representations of the entire anatomy with specific areas for hands, legs, each of our fingers, toes, etc. While there are maps for each body part, there also maps that represent the body as a whole, and the position of body parts in relation to each other at any point of time. The earliest brain map plotted is known as ‘Penfield’s homunculus’ after Wilder Penfield, the physician who led to its discovery. It lies along a narrow strip on the motor cortex less than an inch wide and stretches from ear to ear across the crown of the head, and represents the entire body in the brain. Penfield also found that electrocortical stimulation of the brain invoked four basic types of responses: motor, sensory, interpretive perception, and recall of conscious experience (Penfield 1959). He found that if the temporal lobe was stimulated by an electrode his patients recalled past events. He called the temporal lobe the ‘interpretive cortex’. He was also the first to emphasize the importance of the brain stem (diencephalon) as the seat of consciousness. He wrote:

> There is represented within special areas of the cerebral cortex, special aspects of sensation and special mechanisms of motor control which are indispensable to the individual for an understanding of his environment and for the establishment by him of coordinated action. There is localization also of neurone circuits which seem to be devoted to the recollection of past experience and the interpretation of present perception. But all of these elements would seem to belong to no more than a ‘middle level’ of elaboration in the total function of the brain (Penfield 1947, p. 346).

But later it was found that what Penfield thought to be ‘flashbacks’, or memory recall, were not stored memories. Rosenfield writes:

> Penfield’s discovery suggested to many that we were beginning to uncover the roots of our personalities, our identities, they were eventually to be disillusioned. In the 1970s it became evident that Penfield’s ‘flashbacks’ were not memories at all. The nature of memory and its relation to who we are, our identity remained as mysterious as ever. Careful

> study showed that Penfield had performed similar operations more than one thousand times and that the results were not quite as spectacular as he had hoped. In some ninety percent of his operations the patients failed to have memory flashbacks. He was convinced, however, that he had elicited veridical memories in the ten percent of patients who did have memory flashbacks. But in the 1970s it was discovered that patients only had 'flashbacks' when electrical stimulation of the surface of the brain also affected the limbic system, the part of the brain believed to be essential for emotions. Conscious recollection apparently is not possible without some kind of emotional component. It was furthermore shown that the patients were not recalling events from their childhoods, as Penfield had believed, but were constructing recollections out of observations that they had made on their way to the operating rooms. The patients, however, were convinced that their 'flashbacks' were real memories (Rosenfield 1995, p. 197).

Subsequently, there have been improvements in the representation of the body in the neural cortex and advanced studies on the representation of body and body functions on the neural cortex. A recent report says:

> [T]he areas representing different body parts weren't as well defined as the picture [Penfield homunculus] implies. But new findings go even farther, suggesting that the role of the primary motor cortex might be fundamentally different than originally thought. Rather than simply con- trolling different parts of the body, it might direct a host of body parts to assume complex postures. What's more, the map appears to be organized not just according to muscle groups but by the positions in space where the animal's movements conclude (Helmuth 2002, p. 1587).

Today, neuroscience research tells us that here are several kinds of topographic maps of the body stored in the brain cortex, which are altered and updated according to newer experiences and the changing environment. The brain starts forming maps of the body from early in life. With age and experience our brains would have created and stored several complex maps. Brain maps primarily function as bidirectional feedback systems. Our experiences change the brain maps, and with reorganized brain maps our experiences also are altered.

Apart from the internal and external points of sensation, the body-sense is deeply influenced by certain other mechanisms which are available to us intuitively and without conscious effort. They are the body maps in the brain that make mirror neurons relevant and provide us with proprioceptive capabilities and demarcated peripersonal space. These sensory mechanisms cannot be completely labelled as physical since they involve a collaborative relation with mental attributes. Science is yet to figure out with greater clarity the origins and constituents of body-maps in the brain.

Because of brain maps we have a collection of intuitive, automatic capabilities to perceive location, movement and action of a part of the body in relation with other parts. This group of capabilities is known as proprioception. Proprioception helps us to gauge internally the measure of effort needed to lift and move objects. The measure of effort, of the pressure we exert, is different for lifting or moving different objects. Our body intuitively calculates the precise amount of effort with the help of proprioceptive capability. We are able to take and maintain different postures without falling because of proprioceptive capability. The term 'proprioception', coined by Sir Charles Sherrington (1906), consists of the

Latin *proprius* (one's own) and *perception* and means one's own perception. Sherrington distinguished between senses that are of cutaneous (external), visceral (inner), and deeper (proprioceptive) origin.

Brain maps help us to respond to simple and complex problems, whether they are cognitive or affective. They are continuously updated and reorganized as we live our lives. With the change in our physical disposition, life styles, mental attitudes and emotional responses, brain maps change. The utmost significance of brain maps is indicated by Sandra Blakeslee, a science communicator, in her description of the 'inner self map' (Blakeslee and Blakeslee 2008). We are able to keep track of our movement, position, and sense the extremities of the body with the help of brain maps. There is no one central brain map, but each is unique. The seamless and collective working of body maps in the brain together aid in generating the rich experiences we have and the embodiment we feel continuously without conscious effort. Neuroscience today uses brain maps and mirror neurons that represent the world inside and outside in our brain, to explain emotions, social behaviour, attitudes, etc. If once Crick said, 'our joys and sorrows are a pack of neurons', today the assumption is that our joys, sadness, need to exercise power and all those intricate human tendencies are the result of complex brain maps.

Brain maps are one of the mirroring systems that the brain uses to know 'the other'. Of the mirroring systems the most discussed is the presence of mirror neurons in our brains. Our ability to imitate, learn, empathize, assess the physical and mental condition of the other, to form a theory of mind, all are dependent on mirror neurons present in the mirror systems such as brain maps that influence specific neuronal processes. They are the same class of neurons that become active when we perform an action and when we watch the same action in another person. Interestingly, brain maps not only represent the characteristics of our body but other bodies as well with whom we interact, and they form a shared network. This explains the activity in motor cortex even when we inactively watch someone else performing an activity that we have performed earlier.

The brain maps not only the physical body but also the space around the body, which houses objects, our tools, people with whom we interact, and in short all our socio-cultural expressions. We move around with an arm's length of space around us that we identify as an extension of our body. The space that extends to the limits of our arm or the tip of the tool we use is called the peripersonal space. Peripersonal space is a recently recognized neurological topic. Body-sense is influenced by the peripersonal space we live and move with. Peripersonal space is the invisible volume of space around our body to our arm's length, and it is part of us. My peripersonal space extends to the tip of my pen when I write.

Basically, our peripersonal space is formed of the tools we use, relations we form, dress we wear, houses we live, professions we do, values we hold, beliefs we have, and so on. Our peripersonal space keeps updating as we move and do different things. It continues to include and exclude objects, people and all other entities that come to us in our everyday life. Peripersonal space in a way is an expression of the subjectivity inherent in the body-sense. When I drive a car, my peripersonal space includes the car. The car becomes an extension of my body, and is mapped by the brain accordingly. We include the dress we wear, gadgets we use, beliefs we own, all in our peripersonal space in order to own them as our extensions.

Subjectivity is inherent in the body-sense. The body-sense extends beyond the physical limits of the body as evidenced by the peripersonal space. Through the peripersonal space the brain allows for the inclusion of a major component of our body-sense, which is non-physical. Body becomes more than the biological body by including its psychological, social, and cultural extensions. Peripersonal space integrates our existence in the body, and our extended relation with tools, objects and people. Hence, it also keeps updating itself as we change our ways of behaviour, our beliefs, values, etc. Body-sense is immensely dependent on peripersonal space.

Another way of describing the body-sense is that it is a composite of body-schema and body-image. Body-schema is formed of preconscious, subpersonal processes, proprioceptive and sensory information, because of which movement and maintenance of posture are accomplished (Head 1920) without conscious effort. There are thousands of schemas formed of a lifetime of experience (Arbib 1989). Body-image is the picture that one has of one's own body (Schilder 1950) in one's mind. Body image is also described as a complex set of 'perceptions, attitudes and beliefs pertaining to one's own body' (Gallagher 2005, p. 24) with reflective intentionality. We reflect upon our body image.

5.2.2 Owning Me and My Actions

While the body-senses, proprioception and the brain maps give us a doorway to relate with and know the external and internal worlds, there is another interesting component of the body-sense without which our actions become meaningless. We are the agents of our actions. And, we own our actions. The body-sense comes with the inbuilt capacity for us to sense our actions as ours, and belonging to us. I have a sense of owning my hand, my leg … my body. I am also the agent of my actions. For an action to belong to me, it must be initiated by me and originate from my intentions. Ownership and agency are the twin components of the body-sense that make it compatible for fruitful actions and outcomes.

Can the body-sense be lost, such as in the case of disowning a limb? Today, we know that in subjects with deafferentation, where perceptual or reflective act of consciousness is involved, the self-sense is challenged. Gallagher (2000, p. 15) writes about the patient who was deafferented and deprived of the normal proprioceptive feedback about the position of their limb and could not keep track of it without vision. When the patient was shown a mirror image where a hand was moving, he would say that he was moving his hand, based on the visual cues; when in fact the image was of another person moving his hand. The patient here made a misidentification about who was moving the hand.

Subjects with certain kinds of neurospcyhiatric disorders also are known to disown their own body limbs and thoughts. The Cotard syndrome is where the patient feels that s/he is totally non-existent. Cases of asomatognosia tell us of the varied nature in which the body-sense can be disrupted. Schizophrenic subjects also claim that thoughts have been implanted into their minds and do not belong to them but come from some other source. In such cases, they may have the experience of owning the thoughts, but the sense of agency is affected (Gallagher 2005, p. 174).

Primarily, the sensation of body-absence or disowning a part of the body occurs due to disruption in proprioception and body maps in the brain caused by brain lesions. There is the reverse case such as the phantom limb, where the limb is absent due to amputation but the sense of the limb persists, which again is contributed by the brain's constant attempt to update body maps and utilize neural resources that are no more used. In the former cases, the body part is physically present, but without giving a sense of ownership to the person. And in the case of phantom limb, the sense of the body part continues in spite of its physical absence. Brain maps and proprioceptive capabilities contribute to an intact, coordinated sense of body parts and the body as a whole.

We can say that while the brain is a map-making mechanism, the self is a *meaning-making mechanism*, making sense of what happens to the body, the mind and the environment. Body representations on the brain are continuously updated and reorganized. Body maps become the eye for the brain to see through the million points of the psychosomatic body.[1] Perhaps the brain has acute and extended representation of the minutest nerve and sensory point, in such cases.

5.3 What is the Self-Sense?

Experience is the correlate of the self-sense that comes to our immediate recognition. What are the constituent elements of a typical experience? A typical 'simple' experience (even a visual experience) includes thoughts, sensations, feelings and moods. We may question whether any experience can be marked as 'simplistic'. Even seeing a flower, or hearing a sound, or any such sensation comes with a barrage of memories, desires, feelings, and goals associated with it. Any experience is held tight for the experiencer through a self-concept, which at any point gives an idea of who one is, which acts as the conceptual filter, governs habits and behaviours, and also makes self-transcendence possible. We are able to move from one experience to another or collate different experiences and archive them in memories because of the self-concept. To understand the self-sense is to also see how the self-concept is continually updated or transformed. The self-concept is fed by the 'me and the other' divide, the way we reflect upon ourselves and the other, and our theory of mind, to design our decisions and actions according to assumptions of what the other mind is going through. Two philosophical problems that arise from

[1] For a related discussion, see Zarrilli (2000), who writes about the acutely sensitive body of a master of *Kalaripayattu*, the ancient martial art from Kerala the southern state of India.

the analysis of experience are the inherent subject-object divide; and the amount of the 'other' in 'me', and the 'me' in the 'other'. Are the 'other' and 'me' intrinsically different? What stuff are they made of?

We may have an intuitive sense of the other, but it is very difficult to have a clear, articulated description of oneself. The central problem that underlies the first-person nature of consciousness is the entanglement of the body-sense and the self-sense. Various studies in body-schema and body-image attempt to delineate the body-sense and the self-sense in the first-person experience. It is important to examine both these senses: are they distinct, and if distinct, how? If not, where and how they are entangled? What constitutes these basic, everyday senses? There are fundamental phenomenological and philosophical questions that are absolutely necessary even to attempt such an enquiry. Neurobiology and neuropsychiatry help us ground our questions in matters of experiential concern.

5.3.1 Body Absence and Self-Sense

The larger philosophical question that arises from the curious behaviour of the body-sense is twofold. One, what is that sense which recognizes that there is an absence of the body-sense? Second, what is that sense which feels the sensation of the body part which is physically absent? In other words, how or to whom is the sense of body absence, and the body-sense felt? If we speculate that there is no separate 'who', then we have to concede that body-sense is sensed by the body-sense itself, which is philosophically a redundant position.

Self-sense is an indivisible, continuous and organic, intuitive sense that accompanies human lives. The commonest guideline in biology for assessing the existence of a well-developed self-sense, is the mirror test. Cats and dogs do not recognize their images in the mirror, though they respond to the images. Chimpanzees see the image in the mirror as themselves (marking the chimp with a spot of paint will cause the chimp to touch the marked spot when it sees its image in the mirror). Baboons and macaques fail the mirror test, but they do have a social self. They recognize members of their social group, dominance status, etc.

The self-sense is responsible for self-recognition which makes our lives smooth, comfortable and purpose oriented. It enables us to recognize ourselves as independent entities that exist separate from the environment. I am the thinker of my thoughts, experiencer of my emotions, beholder of my values, attitudes, and owner of all these organically. With the self-sense we become the agents of our bodily movements, possess intentions, make choices, and perform actions. A fundamental feature of the self-sense is the ability to separate the self from others, to recognize oneself as an independent entity that exists distinct from the environment. To make a distinction between changes that happen in the body and in the environment, the self-sense is essential. The self-sense is available to all of us to sense organically. We possess an organic sensitivity. But an accurate description of the most intimate and easily available sense is almost impossible.

The self-sense is challenged by neural impairments and schizophrenia, which also contributes to disruptions in the body-sense. For instance, deafferentation can lead to a reworking of the brain maps and modify representations, owing to cortical plasticity, which leads to phantom phenomena as described by Weir Mitchell in 1871 (Simmel 1958) and Ramachandran (1998). It can also impair proprioceptive capabilities and bodily movements as described by Cole (2004) in *Still Lives*.

It is not easy to exactly describe what we mean, or what we experience as the owner of our body, and our self. Contemporary descriptions such as the narrative self and the autobiographical self indicate this difficulty. Changes in the self-sense happen as a consequence to brain injuries, schizophrenia and spiritual practices. By change I do not mean a change in perspective or attitudes, but fundamental changes that alter self-perceptions and perceptions of the environment.

What is the body of self? What is the (sense of) body? What is the self that is construed by the sense of body, that monitors the body, copes with it, and gives feedback to the self itself? The phenomenology of our subjectivity and ways in which our body-sense and self-sense are represented in our experience is a challenge for neuroscience. Rudrauf and Damasio write:

> Our hypothesis has at least one important limitation in its ability to account for the subjective experience. There is a fundamental and striking phenomenon at the core of subjective experience that it cannot explain: the intrinsic 'spatialization' of our subjective space. We feel in a projective way. The feeling of our own body is a feeling of a body in space, with interoceptive and proprioceptive sensations grossly localized in our extremities and our face. In normal conditions, the 'origin' of the subjective point of view itself feels located or concentrated in our head and perhaps along the main vertical axis of our body. There is really an auto-perceptive structure in which a subjective point of view confronts a set of body states, including itself, in a concrete geometrical space. Such spatialization is a fundamental aspect of the way we build a representation of our body (Rudrauf and Damasio 2005, p. 257).

5.3.2 Bundles, Streams and Technologies of Self

The concept of self is debated as to how and why it is sensed. While Hume described self-sense as 'fluctuating, certain and fleeting' (Smith 1947, p.194), William James suspected that one can never 'catch myself at any time without a perception, and never can observe anything but the perception' (James 1890, p. 351), and Foucault believed that cultures create 'technologies of self' (Foucault 1988).

Hume considered the object and subject aspects of the self-sense as perceptions that occur with inconceivable rapidity and thus give the impression of something that is unchanging. Hume mostly discussed the idea of 'soul' and did not have a distinct theory about the self. He compared the soul to a commonwealth composed of bundles of perceptions that keeps changing. Hume and James held similar views on addressing that function of the self which gives rise to personal identity. Personal identity owes its existence due to resemblance and rapidly changing perceptions. But for James, the self was not just personal identity. His treatment of the self is complex: the components of the self, in his conception, range from the innermost layer to psychological and physical components. James considered consciousness to involve '... a stream of thought, each part of which as 'I' can (1) remember those which went before, and know the things they knew; and (2) emphasize and care paramountly for certain ones among them as '*me*', and *appropriate to these* the rest' (James 1892, p. 215).

Memory and ownership underlie the persistent sense of the self, while the nucleus of the '*me*' is always the bodily existence felt to be present at the time. James sought a layered analysis of the self emphasizing its empirical situatedness. While the material self is constituted by 'bodily appetites and instincts', the social self has the 'desire to please' and to 'be noticed'. James' idea of the 'spiritual self' is perhaps marked by the ideas of the enlightenment period and Kantian theory of moral reason. Spiritual self is marked by 'intellectual, moral and religious aspiration and conscientiousness' (James 1890, p. 329).

From recent times, there are interesting statements on the illusion of a continuous self from Susan Blackmore. She writes:

> [T]he feeling of being a continuous self as an illusion. It is a way of living with what Parfit calls a 'bundle theory' of self as opposed to an 'ego theory' of self. Again and again I seem to be here, to be conscious, to be having a stream of conscious experiences, but I know that this 'me' is just another one of countless 'me's that have arisen and will arise. The apparent continuity of self is not sustained by this 'me' but by the physical continuity of this body and its memories, habits and skills.
>
> More generally, each human body gives rise to a multitude of fleeting selves over its lifetime. These are all somewhat similar because of the continuity of this body with its memories, habits and skills, not because any experiencing self continues. Selves come and go. There may be long gaps with no self, rapid successions of new ones, and even overlapping or simultaneous selves. Mindfulness may maintain a self for long periods, while switches of attention and distractions promote rapid changes. Whenever a self like this is constructed it seems to be having a stream of experiences and easily imagines itself to be the same one who previously experienced the things that this one can now remember, even though this is not true (Blackmore 2012, p. 19).

Is there a deeper core self-sense that is felt? James keeps this question in abeyance and does not commit to a position. He writes:

> ... That (in some persons at least) the part of the innermost Self which is most vividly felt turns out to consist for the most part of a collection of cephalic movements of 'adjustments' which, for want of attention and reflection, usually fail to be perceived and classed as what they are; that over and above these there is an obscurer feeling of something more; but whether it be of fainter physiological processes, or of nothing objective at all, but rather of subjectivity as such, of thought become 'its own object,' must at present remain an open question,—like the question whether it be an indivisible active soul-substance, or the question whether it be a personification of the pronoun I, or any other of the guesses as to what its nature may be (James 1890, p. 304).

James postulates a 'greater Self' which cures the mind, 'giving your private convulsive self at rest', and keeps the discussion open on a core non-reducible self. Such a cure for mind, according to James, though might undermine scientific method its successes can be verified experimentally. He says: 'Such let go helps to be in a world wider than that of world's selfish interest' (1985, p. 111). Further, James develops the ideas of 'healthy-mindedness', 'happiness' and saintliness in his lectures on *The Religion of Healthy-mindedness*, *The Sick Soul* and *Saintliness*, suggesting his interest in considering the self as a core that helps the cure of body-mind from delusions and impairments to personal identity.

According to Wittgenstein, the self-sense is related with first person reference. He proposes two kinds of first person in the famous passage in *The Blue and Brown Book* (1980). The first kind is one that could be mistaken at times: I could go wrong as far as the object of my thought goes. The second kind is one that can be mistaken at no time: The subject of my thought, which is me, the thinker, can never be mistaken to be someone else. For example, if someone says: 'I think there will be a traffic jam today in M.G. Road', they could be wrong about the traffic jam. But they cannot be wrong about the 'I' who thinks about the traffic jam. Following Wittgenstein's classic statement, it will be nonsensical to ask, 'Are you sure that you are the one who is thinking there will be traffic jam?'. The thinker of the thought cannot be mistaken.

> There are two different cases in the use of the word 'I' (or 'my') which I might call 'the use as object' and 'the use as subject.' Examples of the first kind of use are these: 'My arm is broken,' I have grown six inches,' I have a bump on my forehead,'' The wind blows my hair about.' Examples of the second kind are: '*I* see so-and-so,' '*I* hear so-and-so,' '*I* try to lift my arm,' '*I* think it will rain,' '*I* have toothache.' One can point to the difference between these two categories by saying: The cases of the first category involve the recognition of a particular person, and there is in these cases the possibility of an error.... It is possible that, say in an accident, I should feel a pain in my arm, see a broken arm at my side, and think it is mine, when really it is my neighbor's.... On the other hand, there is no question of recognizing a person when I say I have toothache. To ask 'are you sure it's *you* who have pains?' would be nonsensical (Wittgenstein 1980, p. 66).

Shoemaker (2003) describes the first-person subjective reference as 'immunity to error through misidentification'. Self-access is immediate and one does not have to think about it to verify it. He writes:

> The statement 'I feel pain' is not subject to error through misidentification: it cannot happen that I am mistaken in saying 'I feel pain' because, although I do know of someone that feels pain, I am mistaken in thinking that person to be myself.... [T]his is also true of first-person statements that are clearly not incorrigible; I can be mistaken in saying 'I see a canary,' since I can be mistaken in thinking that what I see is a canary or (in the case of hallucination) that there is anything at all that I see, but it cannot happen that I am mistaken in saying this because I have misidentified as myself the person I know to see a canary.
>
> ... If I say 'I feel pain' or 'I see a canary,' I may be identifying for someone else the person of whom I am saying that he feels pain or sees a canary. But there is also a sense in which my reference does not involve an identification. My use of the word 'I' as the subject of my statement is not due to my having identified as myself something of which I know, or believe, or wish to say, that the predicate of my statement applies to it (Shoemaker 2003, p. 8–9).

According to Shoemaker, my access to my-self is immediate and is not dependent on my having to observe it. I do not need to see or reflect on my-self to identify with my-self. For Foucault (1988), the discussion on self is a discussion on technologies of self. Activities such as reading manuscripts, listening to teachers, saying prayers and controlling one's own thoughts and behaviours are techniques by which the self exchanges and updates itself. Technologies of self are devices, according to Foucault, to make possible the social construction of personal identity.

Even before these stalwarts of philosophy, the *Bhagavad Gita*, a few thousand years back, suggested the composite existence of the object and the subject—*kshetra* that which includes the world of the other, and *kshetrajna* that which knows the other (*Bhagavad Gita*, Ch. 13). And, a unique definition to knowledge (*jnana*) in this chapter of the *Gita* is: a set of values that help to see the connections between the 'me' and the 'other'.

5.4 The Range of Self-Sense

In spite of the changes, is there a minimal sense of the self in quadriplegic and paraplegic patients, which remains undisturbed, and with which they cope? In which case what are the features of that minimal self—physiologically, emotionally, cognitively, and also socially, such as values, perceptions, world views, attitudes, values, etc.?

In recent times, the discussion on the self is limited to its function as minimalistic or narrativistic. The idea is to distinguish between a minimal functional self and the self that is continuous over a period of time. While descriptions of self as 'astonishing' (Crick 1995), 'synaptic' (LeDoux 2002), or 'neurochemical' (Rose 2003) are rather straightforward with neural and neurochemical import, the search for a basic, minimal self is not exhausted by a biological concept alone.

Can we derive a very basic self, with basic functions, that still can be called basic? In current discussions, such a basic self is called a minimal self (Gallagher 2000, p. 15). Gallagher elucidates on the 'minimal self':

> Minimal self: Phenomenologically, that is, in terms of how one experiences it, a consciousness of oneself as an immediate subject of experience, unextended in time. The minimal self almost certainly depends on brain processes and an ecologically embedded body, but one does not have to know or be aware of this to have an experience that still counts as a self-experience (Gallagher 2000, p. 15).

The minimal self is what is accessible immediately in a particular moment. It gives the immediate feelings of ownership and agency of action. Agency and ownership are almost indistinguishable in the minimal self. On the other hand, the narrative self has extended functions. We experience ourselves every moment and over a period of time. We remember experiences from the past, and plan for the future. Most importantly, we use words to tell stories and in these stories we create what is called oneself.

A few concepts of the self-sense that are not too minimal or narrativistic are variously termed the 'non-minimal selfy self' and the non-substantial abstract centre of narrative gravity (Dennett 1991); the 'left-hemisphere interpreter' who makes up stories and believes (Gazzaniga 2006); distributed and decentred self (Gallagher 2000); a core, autobiographical self (Damasio 1999). An interesting comparison will be between these concepts and Metzinger's nihilistic concept of 'ego tunnel' (Metzinger 2009) that no one truly possesses. Another provocative view about the self is in comparison with functions such as temperature. Calling self a 'coherence of a personal network', Arbib writes: 'This self is, in my view, no more transcendent with respect to our brains and bodies than temperature is transcendent with respect to molecular motion' (Arbib 2002, p. 175).

Metzinger's concept of the self is provocative in many ways. Firstly, he himself considers his view of the non-existing self as an empirical insight that is 'hopelessly incomplete and necessarily superficial' (Metzinger 2009, p. ix). The gravest error he makes is that he equates what is immediately available to experience with illusion, and he takes a representational schema that produces such an illusion as reality being neurally designed. How can we distinguish an enterprise of modelling which is still an activity that involves human experiences such as thinking and conceptualizing as real, and what it produces as unreal? In the language of a grand illusion, everything has to be the product of that illusion without any relative bias.

Quoting the rubber hand illusion[2] (Botvinick and Cohen 1998), Metzinger equates the feeling (illusorily) experienced as the content of the *phenomenal self-model* (PSM)—the conscious model of the organism as a whole that is activated by the brain (Metzinger 2009, p. 4). Here again, the haste in the argument is seen in equating a particular content or result of an illusion to the illusion of the self-sense itself. That the body experiences tactile sensations referring to an alien limb is not the end of the story of the self's experience. The same self realizes subsequently that such an experience was an illusion. The illusory experience accrues to a self, and the same self subsequently realizes the experience to be illusory. This indicates that there is a core-sense of self which accumulates, updates and distinguishes between the accrued experiences. Without an abiding self, both the initial (illusory) experience and the subsequent realization of it as illusory will not make any sense. Or differently put the question is: for whom is the illusory experience of the 'soul arm' or the 'astral limb' (as mockingly described by Metzinger) and the knowledge of its subsequent illusory nature available?

In his recent book subtitled 'science of mind and myth of self', Metzinger (2009) refers to two illusions to make his central point. The two kinds of illusions that are artificially recreated in laboratory are that of the rubber hand illusion, and the OBE (out-of-body experience) illusion. They illustrate that not only can our bodies falsely identify with alien body parts, but can misidentify another (virtual) body as ours. According to Metzinger, the alien hand is identified as one's own

---

[2] The rubber hand illusion is an experimental illusion examined by Botvinick and Cohen to demonstrate that there is a three-way interaction between vision, touch and proprioception, and that it may supply evidence concerning the basis of bodily self-identification. See (Botvinick and Cohen, 1998, p. 756).

hand because whatever falls in the phenomenal self-model is attributed a conscious sense of ownership and regarded as 'mine'. The brain possesses a whole representation of the body. The sense of self is a 'form of conscious representational content' that can be selectively manipulated under carefully controlled experiments. Self is the representation of the process of representation. It is a 'perspective', according to Metzinger, and the centre of the phenomenal content.

> The PSM of *Homo sapiens* is probably one of nature's best inventions. It is an efficient way to allow a biological organism to consciously conceive of itself (and others) as a whole. Thus it enables the organism to interact with its internal world as well as with the external environment in an intelligent and holistic manner. Most animals are conscious to one degree or another, but their PSM is not the same as ours. Our evolved type of conscious self-model is unique to the human brain, in that by representing the process of representation itself.... We mentally represent ourselves *as* representational systems, in phenomenological real-time. This ability turned us into thinkers of thoughts and readers of minds, and it allowed biological evolution to explode into cultural evolution. The Ego is an extremely useful instrument—one that has helped us understand one another through empathy and mindreading. Finally, by allowing us to externalize our minds through cooperation and culture, the Ego has enabled us to form complex societies (Metzinger 2009, pp. 4–5).

Here, the assumption is that body as a whole and the body parts are the window to experience; experience is the doorway to consciousness; and disruptions in three-way interaction between vision, touch and proprioception can manipulate the self-sense. The mixing up here is between body-sense and self-sense on the one hand, and experience and consciousness on the other. It is argued that embodied consciousness (mind) is real, but non-embodied consciousness is unreal, using the logic of a double-edged sword. The reverse, pointed question would be: how can the unreal self, which is non-existent, accurately describe or know the real and existent bodily experience which is neurally created? Is the brain being taken to be the grand organ that masterminds one's mind, mental life and experiences? Is the singular attention on brain, at the cost of dumping the self, an overrated position? Would considering the brain not as the lone, grand organ but as a 'mediating organ' be a plausible option?

> This mediating role of the brain becomes all the more obvious if we look at it not only cross-sectionally, but include the developmental aspect. The structures of lived experience are inherently mental, i.e. they include spatial, temporal, logical, symbolical, and other patterns which in the course of organism-environment interactions are extracted and ingrained in microstructures of the brain. This results in the formation of neural networks that serve as dispositions for meaningful reactions to similar situations in the future. Thus, in fact *the brain is formed by mental life*; from early childhood on, mental structures come to be imprinted in the brain's structure, and the individual increasingly shapes his own brain through his actions and interactions. The brain may also be regarded as a matrix that transforms all experience into lasting dispositions of behavior and experience (Fuchs 2011, p. 197).

Metzinger and others welcome the 'science of the mind' and dismiss the phenomenal as 'myth'. Self is anathema since it cannot be anything other than yet another feel. The puzzle that Metzinger and friends face is the difficulty in grappling with the phenomenal and the ontological discretely. The puzzle is solved only when it is conceded that the core-self is not another experiential (phenomenal) feel alongside taste, smell, etc., but an ontologically different entity.

5.4.1 Minimalizing the Minimal Self Further

We experience ourselves every moment and over a period of time. There is an extended nature to our self over a period of time. The self is temporally extended. And it is because of the extended temporality of self that we are able to have memories, remember experiences from past, and make plans for the future. The neuropsychological foundation of narrative self is understood from studies on the relevance of episodic memory and disorders with the loss of it affecting normal functioning of the self. The concept of the narrative self was introduced in cognitive sciences by Dennett from psychology, where the narrative and similar ideas about the self are already prevalent (extended, layered, etc.). We use words to tell stories, and in these stories we create what we call our selves. Dennett calls it a 'nonminimal selfy' self.

> There is almost nothing sexy (in human terms) about the sex life of flowers, oysters, and other simple forms of life, but we can recognize in their mechanical and apparently joyless routines of reproduction the foundations and principles of our much more exciting world of sex. Similarly, there is nothing particularly selfy (if I may coin a term) about the primitive precursors of conscious human selves, but they lay the foundations for our particularly human innovations and complications. The design of our conscious minds is the result of three successive evolutionary processes, piled on top of each other, each one vastly swifter and more powerful than its predecessor.... (Dennett 1991, p. 173).

The narrative self is the extended self for psychology. Ulrich Neisser (1988) describes five aspects of the self, based on different forms of information received. These different aspects of the self are rarely experienced as distinct. But they differ in having different developmental histories, aspects of immediacy, and in what they contribute to human experience. They are subject to different kinds of pathologies. The five aspects are: (1) the ecological self—which is directly perceived with respect to the immediate physical environment; (2) the interpersonal self—also directly perceived due to transference of information between members of the species, and through emotional rapport and communication; (3) the extended self—not directly perceived, and based on memory and anticipation; (4) the private self—appears when we discover that our conscious experiences are exclusively our own; and (5) the conceptual self—or self-concept, based on socially based assumptions about ourselves.

The minimalism project for cognitive sciences entails the search for an even more 'primitive' aspect of the minimal self which is not even conceptualized as my-self in an immediate experience. The minimalized minimal self exists even prior to possessing ownership. It is pre-linguistic with non-conceptual elements of the first person. The minimalistic minimal self is the most basic and 'stripped down version' of the self, which can be initiated in an artificial system. But whether human experiences are just behaviours controlled by the brain and cognitive architecture is a valid question to ask. It is not easy, and perhaps not worthwhile, to see human experiences from the lens of artificial systems and robotics.

The crucial factor which is missed in such envision is the human capability to reflect and self-recognize in deeper and organic ways.

Galen Strawson attempts to seek the most basic and stripped down version of the self. According to Strawson, the minimal self is a momentary self without long-term continuity. It is a 'bare locus of consciousness, void of personality', 'stripped of particularity of character, a mere (cognitive) point of view' (Strawson 1997, p. 418). Like in the Buddhist self, the human self is seen to be a collection or series of such momentary selves without continuity. Strawson's minimal momentary self is not restricted to human cases but can be instantiated in non-human animals and robotic systems.

> [I]f one is self-conscious, one must possess the concept (ONE)SELF, and have some conception of experience and of a subject of experience; one must it seems possess the conceptual resources to form and entertain the concept of other subjects; one must be able to think of oneself as a thing or entity in some suitably robust sense; one must be able to identify something as oneself (in the weak sense of 'identify'), and one must possess criteria of subject-identity (where 'criteria' is understood in its conceptual-logical sense) (Shoemaker and Strawson 1999, p. 331).

In contrast, and arguing for a continuous presence, Shoemaker writes about 'paradigmatic embodiment' and how he disagrees with the view that the self is the body, and how each one of us is identical with a 'living human animal'.

> One claim with which I am not sympathetic is that in introspection one is aware of oneself as a body—that one is aware of a body as the subject of one's mental states. If this were true, this awareness would involve an illusion unless we are, in the sense of being identical with, our bodies (Shoemaker and Strawson 1999, p. 288).

According to another theory (Bermúdez 2000), prior to having a sense of the owned self-sense, information is gained in a pre-linguistic and pre-conceptual form from the external environment. According to Gallagher, that such an ecological sense of the self exists can be demonstrated from the capabilities of neonates (less than an hour old) for imitation. Neonates less than an hour old are already able to distinguish between the self and the non-self, use their own body parts proprioceptively, and recognize that the face they see is the same kind as their own (Gallagher 2000, p. 17). The human infant is equipped with a minimal self that is embodied, enactive and ecologically tuned. The idea of the minimal self is the pre-reflective point of origin for action, experience, and thought, according to Gallagher.

However, one significant issue is that even neonates need a primary self-awareness in order to distinguish between the self and the external environment. The theory of the minimal self, which is an ecological self, will face a serious challenge with the question—Won't we need a further 'primitive' self in order to distinguish 'the other' from me?

> This embodied account applies for motor action as well. My actions are not somehow triggered by an inner mind, but they are enacted by me as an embodied subject. When I am writing a letter, for example, there is no point in the unity of action where my 'self' ends and the 'world' begins, no border that separates 'inner' and 'outer world'. Neural

> networks, muscular movements of my hand, pencil and paper synergically work together to put my thoughts down, and the whole body-environment system creates my experience of agency. Being able to write a letter is obviously a capacity not of the brain, but of an embodied subject connected to an environment which provides pencils, paper, words and script. I am not a pure consciousness outside of my own writing, but an '*ecological self*' whose borders do not stop at my skin (Neisser 1988). In the skillful handling of tools, in playing piano or driving a car, I incorporate these instruments. Thus, I feel the paper scratching at the top of the pencil, and being an experienced driver, I feel the roughness of the street below the wheels of my car, just as the blind man feels the ground at the top of its stick, not in his hand. As living bodies, we are extended into the world—always up to the locus where the actual interaction with the world is going on (Fuchs 2011, p. 205).

The greater trouble with the ecological stand of the self is that the baby is thrown out with the bathwater. In the attempt to include the environment, the preponderance of the self in any experience as the fundamental starting point is forgotten. Even to fudge the distinction between the outer and the inner, or to create such a distinction of the 'me and the other', a self that exists in advance before and after the context of the experience is essential. Embodiment theories also face such a challenge. In order for cognitive processes to be embedded in bodily experiences and actions, and for interactions with the environment, firstly a core self-sense is to be conceptualized. The self-sense is not an emergent entity nor one of the cognitive synthesizers, but is fundamental and irreducible.

5.4.2 Why is Minimalism Insufficient?

Why is minimalism insufficient, even if it is complemented by an ecological point of view of the self? It is too minimal to explain the richness of experience, and is inadequate to comparatively discuss the primitive *versus* organic nature of the self. If the 'core-self' postulated by Damasio is continuously reinterpreted, how long can it remain the core? What is that which sustains? If the 'ego tunnel' is non-existent who can vouchsafe for the reality of any experience? By Metzinger's theory, all experiences have to be delusional, since even that entity which gives veracity to experience, the ego, is illusory. What is problematic in discussing a minimalistic minimal self is that experiences of joy, sorrow, etc., are not just 'behaviours' of the brain but complex expressions of the self-sense. Self-sense is the prime motivator of experience and its possibilities. The neural origins are insufficient to explain self-sense.

Damasio in the beginning of his work itself clarifies that he does not go by the argument that consciousness, or the 'necessarily subjective feeling', is an illusion. He writes:

> I shall begin by emphasizing that there is no advantage in considering consciousness as an illusion. The necessarily subjective feeling that we call consciousness is very real, is shared by all of us, writing or reading these words, and it is that reality that requires explanation (Damasio 1998, p. 1879).

A common term used for experience is 'behaviour' in neuroscience. For instance, Dennett writes, we have taken its [consciousness] behaviour (phenomenology) as a 'given' and wondered about what sorts of mechanisms in the brain explain it (1991, p. 171–172). But can our perceptions, joys, feelings, fears and the myriad expressions of self, be just 'behaviours' of the brain? Self-sense, which is a collection of these aspects, or is an 'interpreter', is not just an idea that is explained by seeking its neural origins, but the prime motivator and base of the history and possibility of human experience.

It is not even a resultant of the problem of usage of first-person noun in natural languages. In spite of any language, all human expressions are of a self that is not preconceived by language or a cognitive function. It is a core whose beginnings and range are yet to be ascertained. Damasio writes against the view of consciousness as an emergent property of language acquisition, thus:

> An easy way out on discussions of consciousness is the notion that along with the objective study of behaviors all we need to be concerned with is the study of language, since language might well be the source of consciousness. The idea is that language provides a running commentary on other events of the mind and that human consciousness, in the end, is nothing but that commentary. For a variety of reasons this idea is simply not acceptable. The dependence of consciousness on language would logically rule out the existence of consciousness in any non-human species and in infants. Yet, although one ought to be cautious about commenting on what cannot be observed directly, lucid and comprehensive accounts of the biology of complex non-human creatures suggest that they too are likely to have a basic process of consciousness without which it would be difficult to explain some of the objective behaviors that they exhibit. The notion of language dependence, however, easily runs into an even greater objection. The essence of language coding is the translation of a set of non-verbal representations, that is a 'concept', into linguistic representations, for instance words, signs and sentences. If language were to be the primary source of consciousness, it would have to be true that terms such as 'I' or 'me' would be free-floating novelties that would be the translation of nothing. Of course, that would be a patent absurdity. Terms such as 'I' and 'me', and phrases such as 'I feel pain', are translations of non-verbal concepts that are themselves representative of non-verbal entities and events (Damasio 1998, p. 1880).

The minimal self proposed by neurophilosophers is too minimalistic to explain the rich and complex nature of human experiences. Gallagher's decentred and multiplex, minimal self is a betterment of Dennett's abstract centre, with distributed processing. Damasio calls the minimal self the 'core-self' and the narrative self the 'autobiographical self'. But the core features of the self, as accounted by Damasio, are constantly reinterpreted due to the continuously updated episodic memory and the narrative process. If the core is continuously reinterpreted, how long can it remain the core? Perhaps it is this puzzling question that guides Damasio to suppose that at present the neuroscientist, like the philosopher, can offer an informed speculation, and no well-chartered answers.

Current theories in neuroscience and cognitive science are too reductionistic (either neural or linguistic) and minimalistic in that they have stripped the essential core of the minimal and narrative self. The narrative self, which is reluctantly admitted with many neural and linguistic frills, is also fraught with limits. Gallagher's assumptions about the minimal self is that even if all the unessential features of the self are stripped away, we will still have an intuition that there is a basic, immediate, or primitive 'something' that we are willing to call a self (Gallagher 2000). Gallagher, with much difficulty, concedes to call 'something' a self, which also has to be 'primitive' and 'unessential' and 'immediate'. The central issue of the core-self, which is fully potential, is out of bounds for neuroscience. What comes close to cognitive neuroscience as a viable idea akin to the self is the social brain theory backed up by social cognition and abstractions supported by the 'theory of mind'.

> Concepts such as Theory of Mind, mentalization or simulation all have in common that they conceive of social understanding as implying some kind of inner representations of others' presumed mental states that we then have to project onto them. Research into the 'social brain' has favored a third-person paradigm of social cognition as a passive observation of others' behavior, based upon an inner modeling process in the individual brain. One could even say that according to these concepts the person who perceives another does not actually interact with him or her, but deals with internal models or simulations of her actions (Fuchs 2011, p. 197).

Another theory that comes to the rescue of consciousness being reduced completely to a minimal self is that of Damasio. He distinguishes between two kinds of consciousness, essentially based on the two kinds of memory humans possess—declarative and procedural. However, what Damasio describes as 'core' can be read as primitive, but basic, and present without the intervention of language and memory. And hence, 'core consciousness' is available not just for humans but also other non-human animals. Damasio's core consciousness is not a full-fledged, potential source but a very basic representation constructed by the brain. He writes:

> Core consciousness, or awareness, allows a living organism to sense that the contents of its thoughts are its own, that they are formulated in the perspective of the organism, and that the organism can act on those thoughts. This ability does not rely on language nor does it require great intelligence or memory. Obviously all humans have core consciousness but I shall venture to say that so do individuals of many non-human species. Extended consciousness or consciousness proper surveys a larger canvas of thoughts. Those thoughts portray not just the present state of the organism but also its past and its expected future. They depend on the gradual build-up of an 'autobiographical self', a set of memories of the individual's unique past and expected experiences.
>
> … To put it in other words, how does the organism generate a sense of observer relative to images that are sensed as observed? Without falling into the well-known trap of accounts of consciousness that invoke the homunculus, infinite regress and a central theatre, I have proposed that the answer to these questions requires the understanding of how the brain can build a representation of 'core self' and how knowing is attributed to such a transiently constructed representation. I have suggested that the self is grounded on a representation of the organism, that is, on continuously updated representations of the structure and states of the body. (Damasio 1998, pp. 1880–1881).

The question which is warranted on the discussion of the minimal and the narrative or autobiographical self is: Which is more fundamental and essential—the momentary minimal self, or the extended, autobiographical, narrative self? What is the relation between the minimal self and the narrative self?

Interestingly, it is only because of the presence and conscious intervention of the narrative self, that the functions of the momentary self are corrected in subjects with locomotor disabilities. The subjects Jonathan Cole describes in *Still Lives* (2004), who strive to make some meaning of the motionless and sensationless body, and progress in the quality of their experience in an interactive world, can be understood only if we give place not for a primitive minimal self, but an essential, inclusive, self that guides the functions of the narrative self. To tell a story, a basic, essential, and continuous self-sense is needed. It is minimal in the only sense that it is fundamentally inclusive in nature and underlies the narratives we make of our selves.

Dennett's and Strawson's minimal self is a pre-reflective, pre-intentional self, perhaps also common to all animals. Such a minimal self is dependent on the brain processes and language, and is generated without conscious intervention. Experience happens without the conscious reckoning of the minimal self, which do not extend in time. On the other hand, the narrative self is updated continuously. To facilitate updates and integrate narratives to a whole what is required is an essential (minimal) self. The minimal self has to be a core, ontic self that could be described as non-structured, non-intentional, substantive, pure consciousness.

This leaves us with several questions. Is there a minimal body-sense and self-sense, and according to what criteria? How much of sensation is needed to qualify minimalism? What is the nature of the self-sense? Is it conceptual or experiential? What are the minimal requirements that tell us that we have a self-sense? What are the bodily features of the self-sense? Can we bypass the ethical issues (selves of subjects in vegetative states, and in coma) that emerge from the basic philosophical and biological assumptions about minimal self? According to Strawson, the minimal self can be initiated in a machine, and perhaps switched off and on, since it is mostly the result of interaction between a physical system and the environment. Steven Pinker, the prince of computational theory of mind, believes in reverse engineering to solve the problem of mind. He says:

> I think the key to understanding the mind is to try to 'reverse-engineer' it to figure out what natural selection designed it to accomplish in the environment in which we evolved. In my new book, *How the Mind Works*, I present the mind as a system of 'organs of computation' that allowed our ancestors to understand and outsmart objects, animals, plants, and each other.... What should impress us about the mind is not its rare extraordinary feats, like the accomplishments of Mozart or Shakespeare or Einstein, but the everyday feats we take for granted. Seeing in color. Recognizing your mother's face. Lifting a milk carton and gripping it just tight enough that it doesn't drop but not so tight that you crush it, while rocking it back and forth to gauge how much milk is in the bottom just from the tugs on your fingertips. Reasoning about the world, what will and won't happen when you open the refrigerator door. All of these things sound mundane and boring, but they shouldn't be. We can't, for example, program a robot to do any of them! I would pay a lot for a robot that would put away the dishes or run simple errands, but I can't, because all of the little problems that you'd need to solve to build a robot to do that, like recognizing objects, reasoning about the world, and controlling hands and feet, are unsolved engineering problems. They're much harder than putting a man on the moon or sequencing the human genome. But a four-year-old solves them every time she runs across the room to carry out an instruction from her mother. I see the mind as an exquisitely engineered device: not literally engineered, of course, but designed by the mimic of engineering that we see in nature, natural selection. That's what 'engineered' animals' bodies to accomplish improbable feats, like flying and swimming and running, and it is surely what 'engineered' the mind to accomplish its improbable feats (Pinker 1997).

John Brockman in his introduction to an interview with Pinker, wittingly remarks:

> One of the central metaphors of the third culture is computation. The computer does computation and the mind does computation. To understand what makes birds fly, you

> may look at airplanes, because there are principles of flight and aerodynamics that apply to anything that flies. That is how the idea of computation figures into the new ways in which scientists are thinking about complicated systems. At first, people who wanted to be scientific about the mind tried to treat it by looking for fundamentals, as in physics. We had waves of so-called mathematical psychology, and before that psychologists were trying to find a simple building block—an 'atom'—with which to reconstruct the mind. That approach did not work. It turns out that minds, which are brains, are extremely complicated artifacts of natural selection, and as such they have many emergent properties that can best be understood from an engineering point of view (Brockman 1997).

Here, are we not talking about two completely different scenarios—can there be any serious comparison of the human self or the human mind with artificial systems unless what we are interested is only computational ability?

5.5 Entanglement of the Body-Sense and Self-Sense

Is the self-sense just an inner private sense? It is a composite of experiences, a composite of sensations, emotions and also the ability to exercise free will (even if we concede there is much processing that happens in unconscious levels in the brain). And, more importantly, self-sense entails the 'feeling' of making choices and having control over body. From this perspective, the self-sense is intimately tied with the body-sense. And the reverse also holds true.

The body-sense is always accompanied by a sense of embodiment, of the feeling of having a body and being responsible for its actions. Coupled with ownership and agency, the combined self-sense and body-sense also creates meanings for our actions. We experience those meanings in terms of emotions, values and attitudes, and are the agents of our actions. Can a neural correlate or the brain as a whole be an agent? Philosophically, to attribute functions such as recognition, awareness and agency to the brain, brings in conceptual confusions. In criticism to physicalistic reductionism and psychoneural identity, Jeff Coulter writes: 'Whatever it is that brains do, they do not recognize anything nor do they think of, about or that anything, although they may enable *persons* to do these things' (Coulter 1979, p. 335).

Most of neurobiology studies today is rested on an idea of the entangled body-sense and self-sense. This becomes clearer if we examine the concepts of ownership and agency attributed to the minimal self which has neural origins. The accepted neurological theory is that body ownership and embodiment are the result of information integrated from three sources: vestibular, proprioceptive, and tactile cues (Lopez et al. 2008; Vignemonta 2007).

The greater challenge appears in explaining the ability a deafferented subject who gains neural and motor strength to control the body. For them, the involuntary proprioceptive and motor mechanisms that are available to a normal person is not available. Every thought has to be deliberate and well-planned if it has to lead to a motor action. What is the self-sense in persons whose body-sense is almost completely absent from neck to toe? There is also the reverse case of body-presence and self-absence in the case of trauma due to brain injuries, and in schizophrenia.

Jonathan Cole's (Gallagher and Cole 1998) subjects, due to loss of proprioception and the sense of touch, did not have an intuitive body-sense, but had to look at the body in order to recognize them as theirs. Their body-sense was absent, from neck down, and they were incapable of intentional movement. But by using visual feedback and the intact body-image, some of them, to a limited extent, and over a period of time, were able to control posture and movement. With visual feedback coupled with the sense of body-image, they were able to conceptualize postures and movements. These subjects had to look at their body and think about the body in order to control the body. Multitasking was impossible for them. Their absence of body-image was substituted by the self-sense, a combination of momentary and extended self. Body-sense by any definition was absent. What they had was a mix of self-sense, independent of the body-schema, and the mental *idea* of the body.

How do we explain the self-sense in subjects described by Cole and others, for whom the body-sense is absent? It cannot be dismissed that the body-sense and the self-sense are entangled such that to distinguish them in a clear-cut fashion is almost impossible. Our self-sense and body-sense are intricately intertwined. To separate them distinctly is almost impossible, even in philosophical speculation. Body-sense and the self-sense are rarely available in a discrete fashion to our experiences. Experience comes along with the experiencer and is experienced as a unitary whole. The distinction we make of the entanglement such as body-sense and self-sense is available conceptually (in philosophy) or is available in a laboratory condition where experiments can be designed to manipulate body-identification (for instance, the rubber hand illusion), or in deeper states of focused attention, such as meditation and detached watching.

Once we conceptually examine them as separate, we land upon puzzles of the 'hard problem' type. Aristotle made the famous statement: an unexamined life is not worth having. In a similar vein, perhaps an unexamined self is not worth having. Neurobiology is inspired by the second statement and hence looks for neural origins of qualitative phenomena. Most of neuroscience is based on the premise of consciousness depending on the external world for its manifestation. Since the self-sense is deeply fundamental to all experiences, the mandate of neuroscience is to understand it in terms of its *origins*, and to facilitate a *process* that influences personal identity.

Body-sense and the self-sense are intertwined and share attributes. The core-self is even deeper and is ontically different. When the body-sense is impaired, it is the core-self which is invoked for the recovery of the body-sense. Given the entanglement of self and body-senses, our attempts to understand them distinctly and organically at the same time, also raise entangled questions.

What it is like to live without sensation and movement? If the body cannot sense itself, where does the person reside? Can the self-sense and the body-sense be clearly demarcated in patients incapable of intentional movement, and who have no intuitive body-sense? Figuratively, they have body-absence and self-sense. It is the will and volition that they invoke within themselves, from the cores-self, that help them make some sense of the absence of the body feelings and intuitive capabilities.

It is even conceptually difficult to clearly delineate as to which sense the feeling of making choices and having control over body belongs? Examining them separately, even conceptually, gives rise to a renewed 'hard problem'. The body-sense and the self-sense are intricately intertwined. And at times the self-sense overrides the body-sense, implying that the self-sense has the ability to resort to an undefined, witnessing consciousness for the recovery of the body-sense.

5.6 The Very First Sense

The very first sense that we wake up with is not a sense of the body, but the sense that 'I feel good this morning' or 'I feel bad this morning', or 'I have a muscle cramp that is hurting', etc. Our first sense of the self is also associated with a sense of joy, or peace, or bodily calm. The first moment of self-awareness, if we closely reflect and retrace, is not a thought or a feeling, but a non-conceptual organic sense. It is the 'I-am-ness' that precedes the body-sense and reflexive state of mind that I wish to call as the self-sense. It is fundamental and subliminal in our interactions. However sophisticated our theories of objectifying even the most private feeling, the self-sense is not that which can be known like any other; for the simple reason, that the very moment we try to 'know' and objectify the deeply subjective subject, simultaneously yet another deeply subjective subject would have appeared. The subject 'acts' as if it is diaphanous. The objectification process to convert the subject into an object that can be known brings in another subject *ad infinitum*. The very first sense, the I-am-ness, always stays a subject and without which no knowledge and no experience is possible. But then if again a persistent query is made as to how the subject is known to be the subject without being pervious to the process of knowing, the response offered by ancient philosophers and some contemporary thinkers is that the subject is the light which needs no other light to be illumined. The very first sense of I-am-ness illumines the content of an experience, at the same time being self-luminous.

Is the I-am-ness, or the self-sense, another inner version of the body-sense? The self-sense is not yet another inner sense like the proprioceptive body-sense. The first and last moments of self-awareness are not a thought, or a feeling, but an organic sense. Our self-sense is not a minimalistic sense, but organic and intense at any moment, even for a quadriplegic with proprioceptive challenges. The organic sense cannot be reduced to a minimalistic sense. Hence, the self-sense cannot be cut into parts and a gradient traced from its minimal to extended existence. Or, in other words, the minimalist sense is more a concept and not experientially available. What is present to one's experience is the organic sense which has no minimalist version of it. The self-sense comes as a whole and stays as whole. The self-sense is a continuous *presence*, of what we don't know, and it is not easy to articulate.

In the 10th century AD, Abhinavagupta, the aesthetician from northern India, wrote in his magnum opus *Tantraloka* about the power of the sensation of smell and hearing in invoking deeper aspects of the self, that which touches ones heart. It is difficult and perhaps impossible to verbalize the inner sense that gives shape, form and colour to the content of our experiences. Often, the only way to describe the inner self-sense is by describing the content of the experience. The content of the experience is expected to invoke the 'feel' of the self-sense. Abhinavagupta wrote about the intense sensations that cause vibrations in the self, which is otherwise non-participative. He writes:

> When the ears are filled with the sound of sweet song or the nostrils with the scent of sandalwood, etc., the state of indifference (non-participation) disappears and the heart is invaded by a state of vibration; such a state is precisely the so called power of beatitude, thanks to which human is 'gifted with heart'.(Abhinavagupta, Tantraloka, 3: 200)[3]

In a similar vein, Gerards Manley Hopkins, a nineteenth century Jesuit priest and Victorian poet, uses the sensation of taste to describe the essence and intense feeling of the self. He writes:

> When I consider my self-being, my consciousness and feeling of myself, that taste of myself, of *I* and *me* above and in all things, which is more distinctive than the taste of ale or alum, more distinctive than the smell of walnut leaf or camphor, and is incommunicable by any means to another man.... Nothing else in nature comes near this unspeakable stress of pitch, distinctiveness, and selving, this self being of my own. (Hopkins, quoted in Manoussakis 2007, p. 51)

For both Abhinavagupta and Hopkins, the very first moment of self-recognition itself is plenitude, a state of vibration, and does not need anything further for its existence. The self-sense like any other sensation is intense, felt at once, and does not need a via media. But the difference between other sensations and the self-sense is that the rest of the sensations get a place, meaning and adherence only in the light of the self-sense.

An existentialist philosopher like Sartre also liked to believe in a self-sense that is intense, and a self that has to choose between 'either-or'. But for Sartre, it is nausea, and not a taste, that the organic sense of the self generates.

5.7 A Proposal

Advances in neuropsychiatry and neurophenomenology, and the continuing interest in neurophilosophy, inspire us to find the limits of the larger questions we raise, and from there on how we can extend the limits conceptually. To what extent can science study the self-sense? How much or what parts of it are amenable for

[3] tatha hi madhure gite sparse va chandanadike madhyathi avagameya sauhrdaye spandanamanata anandasaktih saivoktayatah sahrdayoh janah (Abhinavagupta, Tantraloka 3:200).

empirical enquiry? Are we short sighted in our imagination to conceptualize the self dynamically and organically while we label it as a neuropsychological process, a narrative creation, or an emergent property that can be simulated in artificial systems? Is the self essentially private and subjective? Does the essentially private nature of the self make it non-existent conceptually when we theorize experience and consciousness?

Often our discussion on the self is limited to the waking state, while we also know that consciousness deeply impinges upon our personhood by our capacities to reflect, meditate, dream and sleep. Hence, it is all the more important to understand the influence of these states in the waking state and thereby the self-sense. Studies in pathologies that affect the body-sense such as schizophrenia and identity disorders make it imperative for us to ponder upon both the unstable and stable elements that are expressed through the self-sense. Cultural neuroscience reminds us how much of our worlds are shared and intersubjective; how much of the self is the body-sense, and how much of it is not dependent on the body-sense; and that there is a sense of self in bodies with deafferentation and minimal proprioception.

The self-sense has two aspects that are mutually irreducible, but cannot be conceptually delineated completely from one another. The self-sense is immediately accompanied by the body-sense. The body-sense is immediately accompanied by the self-sense.

The self-sense, we could say, can be understood in terms of three basic senses:

1. The outer sense of the self in relation with the environment, generated by brain maps, proprioceptive capabilities (movement, posture) and sensations, that extends beyond the body to its peripersonal space (thus, the body is no more a physical entity, but a cultural, social, spiritual entity);
2. the inner sense with an essential core, but continuous, existing every moment and extending temporally; and,
3. the innermost organic core-self, which is trans-spatiotemporal, which wisdom traditions describe as pure consciousness—an unstructured realm of possibilities.

The concepts we use to analyse human experiences have witnessed intense debates spanning centuries. While the humanities (religion, arts, literature, and philosophy) almost always use free flowing narratives, social and natural sciences look for simple building blocks that can be manipulated in order to explain the origins of complex phenomena. A similar contribution is made by the psychoanalytic and social cognitive approaches to the self, resulting in constant questioning of the very existence of the self.

> The first limitation of psychoanalytic accounts is equally a problem for social-cognitive theories-namely, a lack of conceptual and semantic clarity, leaving many observers with the impression that 'the self' is a mushy, muddle-headed construct without empirical referents. Theorists of every persuasion consistently use the terms self and self-schemas or self-representations interchangeably, leading to persistent questions about what is being represented and what the boundaries of this construct could be. Further, both cognitive

> and psychoanalytic theories tend to include more and more phenomena in their quasi-definitions of self, rarely noting the change in the construct, and ultimately including almost anything of any psychological importance under the rubric (Westen 1992, p. 4).

Thanks to the polar division in the approach to human experiences (one, self-actualization, and the other, self-naturalization), a balance is often reckoned whenever extreme positions are maintained. We need to explore the self-sense multidirectionally—biologically, psychologically and spiritually. Both the first-person and the third-person approaches are needed. But in both the very core of the self-sense has to be included non-reductively and at the same time in non-abstraction.

One of the suggestions for reconciliation is to bring in the *whole person* side by side with the discussion on cognitive structures such as the self-schema.

> The only consistent use of the term self is to use it as in colloquial speech, to refer to the person (as in herself or myself). This permits a logical definition of self-schemas or self-representations as mental representations of the self, that is, of the person (Westen 1992, p. 7).

We also have to be guided by larger questions that seek long-term human welfare and wellbeing. From that point of view, will the trend for extracting a minimal self pay off? How much of sensation is needed to call the self-sense minimal? What is the sense of self in bodies with spinal cord injuries and those that have limited or no proprioception? Can the self-sense that ensues (if it does) from brain-maps tell us what is distinctive about it? How much of the self is in the other? How much of the self is in the body-sense? How much of it is not dependent on the body-sense? And, most importantly, how much of the self is amenable to neurobiological enquiry?

I wish to make an assumption. Just as brain is a map-making mechanism (representations of body, its environment—physical, psychological and cultural), is self a *meaning-making* 'mechanism', that helps us to make sense of everything else around and within? Because, even if cognitive neuroscience might do away with the 'self-sense' by theorizing its absence causally (neural behaviour) and functionally (information networks), still the core of the self-sense will persist organically in our actual everyday experiences. There is a persistent organic wholeness in every experience. How does neuroscience understand the organic wholeness? Is it an observable, empirical phenomenon?

> When a biologist looks at or listens to or palpates a human body he encounters various anatomical entities and functional relationships. For a long time systematic study of these objective realities provided the principal scientific base for the practise of medicine. As the biologist employs more and more refined instruments, he sees smaller and smaller details and, by resorting to chemical methods, he can infer even morphological elements and the functional relations between them. But no matter how closely he looks, or how refined his chemical methodology, he does not encounter any empirical reality resembling what other people have in mind when they talk about personhood. Failing to discover personhood among observable biological facts, he might look next for what may be inferred from other facts. As one pokes in this area, one soon encounters the notion that a whole organism acts as if it were more than the mere sum of its parts. Since personhood implies a similar transcendence it seems reasonable to look for some relation between it and a hypothetical 'wholeness factor' (Morison 1983, p. 4).

Even the 'minimal self' and 'computational mind' hypothesis are postulated by a self, a person, who has likes and dislikes, preferences and priorities. There is no value-free neural self at any time except in the pages of a book, or the theory behind an experiment, as a concept. Whether we like it or not, the self-sense comes to us not as a neutral and bland self but as a rich whole permeating the entire being at the very first moment itself. We might conceptually get rid of a rich whole, organic, self-sense. But can we do away with such a 'self-sense' experientially? Impossible!

References

Arbib, M. A. (2002). In: M. Richardson, R. J. Russell, P. Clayton, & K. Wegter-McNelly (Eds.), *The horrors of humanity and the computation of the self.* London: Routledge.

Arbib, M. A. (1989). *The metaphorical brain 2: Neural networks and beyond.* New York: Wiley-Interscience.

Bermúdez, J. L. (2000). *The paradox of self-consciousness: Representation and mind.* Cambridge: MIT Press.

Blackmore, S. (2012). She won't be me. *Journal of Consciousness Studies, 19*(1–2), 16–19.

Blakeslee, S., & Blakeslee, M. (2008). *The body has a mind of its own: How body maps in your brain help you do (almost) everything better.* New York: Random House.

Botvinick, M., & Cohen, J. (1998). Rubber Hand 'Feels' Touch That Eyes See. *Nature, 391*, 756.

Brockman, J. (1997, November 1). *Organs of computation: A talk with Steven Pinker.* Retrieved 28 June 2012, from Edge Third Culture: http://www.edge.org/3rd_culture/pinker/pinker_p1.html.

Cole, J. (2004). *Still lives: Narratives of spinal cord injury.* Cambridge: MIT Press.

Coulter, J. (1979). The brain as agent. *Human Studies, 2*(4), 335–348.

Crick, F. (1995). *The astonishing hypothesis: The scientific search for the soul.* New York: Simon & Schuster.

Damasio, A. (1999). *Feeling of what happens: Body and emotion in the making of consciousness.* London: Heinemann.

Damasio, A. R. (1998). Investigating the biology of consciousness. *Philosophical Transactions: Biological Sciences—The Conscious Brain: Abnormal and Normal, 353*(1377), 1879–1882.

Dennett, D. (1991). *Consciousness explained.* London: Allen Lane.

Dennett, D. (1996). Facing backwards on the problem of consciousness. *Journal of Consciousness Studies, 3*(1), 4–6.

Foucault, M. (1988). In L. H. Martin, H. Gutman, & P. H. Hutton, (Eds), *Technologies of the self.* Massachusetts: University of Massachusetts Press.

Fuchs, T. (2011). The brain—A mediating organ. *Journal of Consciousness Studies, 18*(7–8), 196–221.

Gallagher, S. (2005). *How the body shapes the mind.* Oxford: Oxford University Press.

Gallagher, S. (2000). Philosophical conceptions of the self: Implications for cognitive science. *Trends in the Cognitive Sciences, 4*(1), 14–21.

Gallagher, S., & Cole, J. (1998). *Body and flesh: A philosophical reader.* In D. Welton, (Ed.) Oxford: Blackwell.

Gazzaniga, M. (2006). *The ethical brain: The science of our moral dilemmas.* New York: Harper Collins.

Head, H. (1920). *Studies in neurology* (Vol. 2). London: Oxford University Press.

Helmuth, L. (2002). Redrawing the brain's map of the body. *Science, New Series, 296*(5573), 1587–1588.

James, W. (1892). *Psychology.* New York: Henry Holt and Company.

James, W. (1890). *The principles of psychology.* Retrieved 7 April 2012, from Classics in the History of Psychology: http://psychclassics.asu.edu/James/Principles/prin10.htm.
James, W. (1985). In M. E. Marty (Ed.), *The varieties of religious experience: edited with an introduction.* New York: Penguin Classics.
LeDoux, J. (2002). *Synaptic self: How our brains become who we are.* New York: Penguin Books.
Lopez, C., Halje, P., & Blanke, O. (2008). Body ownership and embodiment: vestibular and multisensory mechanisms. *Clinical Neurophysiology, 38*, 149–161.
Manoussakis, J. P. (2007). *God after metaphysics.* Bloomington: Indian University Press.
Metzinger, T. (2003). *Being no one: The self-model theory of subjectivity.* Cambridge: MIT Press.
Metzinger, T. (2009). *The ego tunnel: The science of the mind and the myth of the self.* New York: Basic Books.
Morison, R. S. (1983). Is there a biological person? *The Milbank Memorial Fund Quarterly: Health and Society: Special Issue: The Problem of Personhood: Biomedical, Social, Legal and Policy Views, 61*(1), 3–18.
Neisser, U. (1988). Five kinds of self-knowledge. *Philosophical Psychology, 1*(1), 35–59.
Penfield, W. (1947). Ferrier lecture: Some observations on the cerebral cortex of man. *Proceedings of the Royal Society of London. Series B, Biological Sciences, 134*(876), 329–347.
Penfield, W. (1959). The interpretive cortex. *Science, New Series, 129*(3365), 1719–1725.
Pinker, S. (1997, November 1). *Organs of computation: A Talk with Steven Pinker.* In J. Brockman (Ed.) Retrieved 28 June 2012, from Edge Third Culture: http://www.edge.org/3rd_culture/pinker/pinker_p2.html.
Ramachandran, V. (1998). *Phantoms in the brain.* New York: William Morrow.
Rose, N. (2003). Neurochemical selves. *Society, 41*(1), 46–59.
Rosenfield, I. (1995). Memory and identity. *New Literary History: Narratives of Literature, the Arts, and Memory, 26*(1), 197–203.
Rudrauf, D., & Damasio, A. (2005). A conjecture regarding the biological mechanism of subjectivity and feeling. In G. Colombetti, & E. Thompson (Eds.) *Journal of Consciousness Studies, 12*(8–10), 236–262.
Schilder, P. (1950). *The image and appearance of the human body.* New York: International Universities Press.
Searle, J. R. (1997). *The Mystery of Consciousness.* New York: The New York Review of Books.
Shear, J. (1996). The hard problem: Closing the empirical gap. *Journal of Consciousness Studies, 3*(1), 54–68.
Sherrington, C. S. (1906). *The integrative action of the nervous system.* New Haven: Yale University Press.
Shoemaker, S. (2003). *Identity, cause, and mind: Philosophical essays.* Oxford: Oxford University Press.
Shoemaker, S., & Strawson, G. (1999). Self and body. *Proceedings of the Aristotelian Society, Supplementary Volumes, 73*, 287–332.
Simmel, M. L. (1958). The conditions of occurrence of phantom limbs. *Proceedings of the American Philosophical Society, 102*(5), 492–500.
Smith, N. K. (Ed.) (1947). *Dialogues concerning Natural Religion* 2nd edition, Edinburgh: Nelson & Sons.
Strawson, G. (1997). The self. *Journal of Consciousness Studies, 4*(5–6), 405–428.
Vignemonta, F. D. (2007). Habeas corpus: The sense of ownership of one's own body. *Mind and Language, 22*, 427–449.
Westen, D. (1992). The cognitive self and the psychoanalytic self: Can we put our selves together? *Psychological Inquiry, 3*(1), 1–13.
Wittgenstein, L. (1980). *The blue and brown book.* New York: Harper & Row.
Zarrilli, P. B. (2000). *When the body becomes all eyes: Paradigms, discourses and practices of power in kalarippayattu, a South Indian martial art.* Oxford: Oxford University Press.

Chapter 6
Boundaries of Self: Displacement, Meaning and Purpose

Even while you say there is no self, you need food when you feel hungry; you need respect; you need love. Our intellectual beliefs and experiences seem to be different. The spirit in the human to survive and live happily cannot be suppressed by anyone. The self that is revised or destroyed is our idea of the self; only our concepts of the self are revised or destroyed.

Swami Bodhananda in conversation with the author, 2005.

Running through every single experience, whether it is the casual and routine sipping of coffee, or a complex one of creative joy, or loving someone, are various emotions, memories and decision-making processes. The self gives unity to discrete components, binds them to the experiencer, and makes them meaningful. The self is the single unit of information and experience, which provides adherence for various experiences extended in time.

The self presents to us meaningful experiences. Without a self, there is no experience that is lived. Without the self, experience is just archived information. Self is the subjective unit that connects and presents complex information in a discrete but interconnected manner. In spite of the abstruse technical concepts that connect the self with neural mechanisms, we feel at home with the self since it is close to our very existence, giving meaning to silly and serious things we do in life. The self's interest is to make sense of what is around and what is presented.

What do we mean by 'meaning' of experience?

Is there a body-mind and brain-self continuum that contributes to the attribution of meaning?

Mostly, in an experience, we focus on the cognitive content coupled with the role of agency and action. Further, such a focus results in a schismatic view of the person as a whole, and the person in a discrete moment with certain sensory-motor and cognitive functions.

S. Menon, *Brain, Self and Consciousness*, Studies in Neuroscience, Consciousness and Spirituality, DOI: 10.1007/978-81-322-1581-3_6,

At any time, you and I are endowed with personhood as a whole which is a combination of beliefs, attitudes, approaches, preferences, dispositions, emotions, values, insecurities, desires, expectations, and a purpose for life and living. Once we isolate a particular cognitive or sensory-motor function from the personality of the person as a whole, we can no more talk about the person, but only about the particular function, which is depersonalized.

I would say that the meaning of an experience is the value given to that experience in responding to it in terms of a physical and mental action, attitude, emotive valence, memory evoking, consequential thinking, and value system, all assimilated to contribute to the formation of purpose. Every experience leaves a mark from the past and carries forth a mark to the future. It is our ability to move forward with expectations and plans for the future that gives directions to the purpose, finally making an experience meaningful. Without meaning there is no purpose. And without purpose, meaning has no sustenance.

Every experience contributes to the purpose of living in the body and the mind. But the realm of perceiving the purpose and thereby creating a meaning itself need not be the result of sensory and cognitive capabilities, but the result of our innate relation with the inner core-self that can be identified with a space of infinite possibilities.

6.1 Tracing the Contours of Self

Experiences tell us that the boundaries of the self-sense are flexible, contributing to better or worse existences. The self at times can be fractured or become fragile. The self for some people is the most encompassing and inclusive phenomenon, leading to self-actualization. Nevertheless, that the boundaries shift is no evidence for establishing that there is no self. All the while in and through different experiences an overall value of the self-sense stays, which carries forward the agenda of seeking purpose and thereby achieving meaning. There is a continuity in all our experiences which brings forth the past, present and future to the same moment.

We are capable of thinking using information from the past and expectations about the future. Memories are closely connected and contiguous to all our experiences. Such continuity is felt as adhering to a single unit of consciousness which we call my-self. Contrary to the Cartesian dictum ‘I think, therefore I am’, in our daily life we first *are*, and therefore are able to do many things, mental and physical. Otherwise all our physical and mental acts will not have a place to adhere to and will be floating around.

We are able to give interconnected meanings to our experiences, learn from mistakes, form beliefs, cherish hopes, have insecurities, express emotions, reflect upon the *faux pas* we make in life—all these rich forms of experiences, with an unwavering unity and coherence. The first and foremost features of the self are: being (to put it more experientially, the ‘I-am-ness’), continuity, adherence, coherence and unity. All through these several features of the self at any point we are capable of different degrees of awareness and reflection.

Perhaps in the evolutionary scale what marks the human self as distinct is our capacity to be self-aware in multiple and deeper levels. Our hidden capabilities for complex levels of awareness and reflection are amply dealt with in the Eastern traditions, to mention a few—the concept of *samyama* in Patanjali's *Yogasutras*, *sakshi-caitanya* in Vedanta, *sthitaprajna* in the *Bhagavad Gita*, and *rasa* in the *Natyasastra*.[1]

6.1.1 Brain Impairments and Body Displacements

Ramachandran, in his five-list attributes for self (2003, pp. 113–114), talks about embodiment, agency and the ability to be self-aware as important features of the self. We have a sense of belonging or ownership to the body. We exercise free will. We self-reflect. However, centuries have passed by since the connections between matter and consciousness, the body and the self are debated with unflinching vigour but with no clear solution to comprehend the nature of this relation.

The boundaries of the self seem to shift and shrink in the case of the narratives neuropsychiatrists mention about brain impairments. Brain impairments are caused by lesions—damage or removal of brain areas—as a result of stroke or surgery. The self's capability for expansion and non-dual inclusion seems to be vital for Vedantic and other spiritual traditions. Both neuroscience and spiritual traditions, give *mindboggling* accounts of challenges and possibilities for the self, literally and figuratively. And, also what is acknowledged in both accounts is the recognition of the mutual challenge between the body and the spirit, the brain and the self. Let us look at some of the curious challenges the brain can give to the self, and the self to the brain, causing disturbances to our otherwise natural intuition for proprioception—the feeling and knowledge of the position of the body in space.

With a novel-like quality, Ramachandran and Blakeslee (1998), Ramachandran (2003), Feinberg (2001), Damasio (1999, 2003), Sacks (1985), Cytowic (2002) and others narrate strange and unthinkable experiences, and traverse through the mind of the patient like a detective to find the route to the cause that generates the 'irrational' behaviour. The dialogue between the patient and the doctor itself in these narratives provides a wonderful opportunity for readers to get insights about two selves—an impaired one that is being treated, and another intact one attempting to set right the impaired one.

Let us look at a few cases of brain impairments where the self struggles without giving a clue for theories and arguments to make sense of it. The human self in these cases appears to be quite fragile and prone to the changes in neural circuitry.

[1] For a discussion on the text, see Sastri and Nagaraja Rao (1990).

In the case of *phantom limb*, patients are aware that the phantom limb is physically absent, but experience the pain that originates from it. Ramachandran writes the case of one of his patients:[2]

> Tom was not crazy. His impression that his missing arm was still there is a classic example of a phantom limb—an arm or leg that lingers indefinitely in the minds of patients long after it has been lost in an accident or removed by a surgeon. Some wake up from anesthesia and are incredulous when told that their arm had to be sacrificed, because they still vividly *feel* its presence. Only when they look under the sheets do they come to the shocking realization that the limb is really gone. Moreover, some of these patients experience excruciating pain in the phantom arm, hand or fingers, so much so that they contemplate suicide. The pain is not only unrelenting, it's also untreatable; no one has the foggiest idea of how it arises or how to deal with it (Ramachandran and Blakeslee 1998, p. 21).

Prosopagnosia is generalized disturbance in face recognition. Patients with prosopagnosia are unable to identify anyone by looking at their faces. Prosopagnosia, in severe cases, impairs self-recognition in the mirror and also destroys common intuitions such as the immediacy of self-awareness.[3]

Asomatognosia is a condition where one's own paralysed limbs are misidentified for someone else's. The severe form of this impairment is *anosognosia*, where the paralysis or the illness is ignored or denied. Feinberg (2001, p. 17) cites the work of the neurologist Edward Weinstein who argues that the manner in which asomatognosia patients refer to their arms as belonging to someone else could be interpreted as metaphorical expressions of their feelings about themselves. He held that patients with asomatognosia who misidentified parts of their body displayed a disturbance in metaphorical speech and tended to express their feelings about themselves metaphorically.

In these and other cases, brain continuously creates meaning and projects the self in that context though it might appear irrational for the onlookers. Feinberg states that in spite of the brain impairment, the use of metaphorical language demonstrated by these patients served to bring order, unity, and predictability to the frequently confusing circumstances of neurological illness. The self somehow helps to cope with the brain challenge and create a corresponding meaning and integrated sense of what happens. Feinberg says:

> One of the interesting aspects of asomatognosia is that, despite the fragmentation of the self, these patients strive to maintain an integrated self and make sense of their experience. Indeed, to a large extent they succeed. The neglected left side and the misidentified

---

[2] In his book *Phantoms in the Brain* (1998), Ramachandran brings in fascinating information about Penfield maps. These maps, drawn by the Canadian neuroscientist Wilder Penfield, in the 1940s and 1950s, show that the whole body is represented on the surface of the brain. The brain representation is disproportionate, with some of the body areas represented in large parts of the brain, like mouth, palm and feet, and some in small areas, like the body trunk. Ramachandran, with his work on phantom limbs, shows that striking reorganizations in body image occur very rapidly following the amputation of a limb. Phantoms limbs are generated by such reorganizations of body image in the sensory cortex. Also See Sect. 5.2.1 in Chap. 5.

[3] For details, see Ramachandran and Blakeslee (1998), Feinberg (2001).

left limb leave a hole, a gap, in the self, that must be filled. The patient may disavow the arm, but something is put in its place, something of personal significance (Feinberg 2001, p. 30).

Hemispatial neglect is the condition where objects and one's own body parts on one side of the body (on the side opposite a brain lesion, usually left side) are neglected. Patients with hemispatial neglect do not simply ignore stimuli on one side but act in a manner as if nothing of personal significance could occur on that side (Feinberg 2001, p. 13). If they are asked to draw a daisy it is drawn with the left side incomplete. They ignore food on the left side of the plate while having a meal. Neglect patients are profoundly indifferent to objects and events on the left side of the world, sometimes including the left side of their own bodies (Ramachandran and Blakeslee 1998, pp. 82, 88). Hemispatial neglect is severe and long lasting after damage to the right hemisphere, according to Feinberg's studies.[4] Asomatognosia, hemispatial neglect and anosognosia often occur together, usually as a result of damage to the right hemisphere.[5]

Capgras' and *Cotard's syndrome* are cases where patients are unable to give an emotional reference to what they see because of disruptions in brain circuitry between the eye (or all sense organs) and the emotional centre.[6] In the case of

[4] See Feinberg (2001, p. 12): 'The right hemisphere has the capacity to direct attention to both sides of space. When there is damage to the left hemisphere, the right hemisphere can compensate for the loss, and the patient is still aware of both sides of the world and the self. On the other hand, the left hemisphere is much more unilateral in its attentional capabilities, and is best at directing the patient's attention to the opposite (right) side. In the presence of damage to the right hemisphere, the left hemisphere has limited capacity to adapt, and the left side of space and the body may be ignored'.

[5] Feinberg (2001, p. 22) narrates the case of Jack: 'Jack had asomatognosia and misidentified his left arm. He also had dense anosognosia and insisted that he was in pretty good health. He made this claim, even though he was lying in a hospital bed in a gown, with an intravenous line in his right arm. Jack knew, all too well, that the doctors thought he was ill, that he had suffered a stroke; he even knew the hospital staff thought he could not move his left side. Despite this knowledge, he held to his belief that he was not ill in any way. Jack insisted that all was well…'.

[6] See Ramachandran and Blakeslee (1998, p. 116): 'A better approach for studying Capgras' syndrome involves taking a closer look at neuroanatomy, specifically at pathways concerned with visual recognition and emotions in the brain… the temporal lobes contain regions that specialize in face and object recognition… We know this because when specific portions of that pathway are damaged, patients lose the ability to recognize faces, even those of close friends and relatives—as immortalized by Oliver Sacks in his book *The Man Who Mistook His Wife for a Hat.* In a normal brain, these face recognition areas (found on both sides of the brain) relay information to the limbic system, found deep in the middle of the brain, which then helps generate emotional responses to particular faces… I may feel love when I see my mother's face, anger when I see the face of a boss or a sexual rival or deliberate indifference upon seeing the visage of a friend who has betrayed me and has not yet earned my forgiveness. In each instance, when I look at the face, my temporal cortex recognizes the image—mother, boss, friend—and passes on the information to my amygdala (a gateway to the limbic system) to discern the emotional significance of that face. When this activation is then relayed to the rest of my limbic system, I start experiencing the nuances of emotion—love, anger, disappointment—appropriate to that particular face…'.

Capgras' syndrome, the patient comes to regard close acquaintances—usually one's parents, children, spouse or siblings—as impostors (Ramachandran and Blakeslee 1998, p. 115). In Cotard's syndrome, the patient will assert that he is non-existent and dead. Ramachandran and Blakeslee argues (1998, p. 119) that Cotard's syndrome is an exaggerated form of Capgras' syndrome and probably has a similar origin. In Capgras' syndrome, the face recognition area alone is disconnected from the amygdala. In Cotard's syndrome, all the sensory areas are disconnected from the limbic system, leading to a complete lack of emotional connect with the world.

In these cases of strange self-ascriptions, what strikes us is the self's capacity to make meaning of what is experienced, even while the brain circuitry is severely severed. The person is seen, but no emotion is invoked towards the person seen. But since the brain 'sees' the person, the self-sense has to find some meaning and associate relevance to what is seen. Hence, the patient connects emotionally (without the corresponding circuitry to the visual area) and identifies the person seen as an impostor. As Ramachandran succinctly says (1998, p. 116), with the disruption in the neural circuitry between the visual and the emotional areas, the patients need to only see a face that is not familiar. Why should s/he impute the meaning of an impostor? The possible answer to this question is that the self perhaps constantly tries to solve dilemmas even when they are neurally created.

Are meaning-giving and unification of experiences functions of the brain or the self? We may argue either way. I would like to think that it is the core-self (not in the sense of Damasio's 'core consciousness'), the deeper and complex realm of our being, which is not pervious to our methods of knowledge, that helps generate meaning, because meaning is a value with implications for a lasting existence. It can be related with the ontology of the core-self qua pure consciousness.

The reason that often discussions on the self take a reductive pattern is the general assumption that consciousness is primarily 'sensory awareness'—awareness of a sensation. Therefore, the focus of discussion is on implicit perceptions and similar phenomena. But, to equate consciousness to one functional aspect will be to equate the sea with one drop of the sea water, and to foreclose the potential and possibility of the self.

6.2 Self-Recognition and the Core-Self

Self-recognition and recognizing the other are the two prominent parameters for ascertaining self-concept. Variables that consider different functions and degrees of self-recognition and other-recognition are used in experiments designed by cognitive neuroscience to measure the self and find its place in the brain. The basic function that underlies self-recognition is considered to be 'self-awareness'. There are mainly two views about the neural origin of self-awareness, according to a recent study which distinguishes between three levels of self-awareness such as core, extended and introspective (Philippi and Feinstein 2012). One view is that specific brain regions such as anterior cingulate cortex, medial pre-frontal cortex and insula are responsible for the origin of self-awareness, while the other view is that distributed cortical and sub-cortical networks are responsible for self-awareness. Studies based on anosognosia[7] of hemiplegia that result in impaired self-awareness reveal that normal self-awareness is dependent on several parallel processes.

> One must have sensory feedback and the ability to attend to both one's body and the space where parts of the body may be positioned or acting. One must develop a representation of the body, and this representation must be continuously modified by expectations (feed-forward) and knowledge of results (feedback) (Heilman et al. 1998, p. 1903).

What these studies indicate is that today neuroscience mostly takes self-awareness and self-recognition as a composite and as neurally located.

Functional and structural approaches backed by developmental psychology, to a certain extent, help frame possible causes for challenges faced in pathologies that impair self-perceptions and social interactions. But to ascribe the self itself as located in the brain implies a poor conceptual grounding.

The complexity, richness and the ontological primacy of the self are understood to a large extent once we analyse the content of its recognition. No doubt, the self recognizes. And the most accepted empirical feature of recognition is self-image. The test of recognizing the self's image on the mirror has been the original step to describe consciousness as bidirectional (Gallup 1977) enabling awareness of the outside world, and self-awareness.

To ascribe recognizing one's self-image as the indicator for possessing consciousness—though an important criterion—is a problematic assumption when we consider the self-sense of subjects who fail to recognize their faces and others' due to neurological impairments. At the same time, the tendency to state that introspection on one's mental states is not a good enough indicator of consciousness needs review. According to Zahavi, the phenomenological method involves reflection that is prior to the divide of the exterior body and the inner mind (Zahavi 1999, 2005, 2011). For Zahavi, reflection and introspection have different focus. Michel Bitbol clarifies on the essential introspective nature involved in reflection, and disagrees with the contention that the reflecting and the reflected face each other. He writes:

> Reflection does not amount to perceiving consciously some unconscious event taken as an object (unlike Freud in his *Papers on Metapsychology*), but rather renewing contact with experience and defocusing/refocusing our attention (Bitbol and Petitmengin 2011, p. 25).

Recognizing oneself involves complex levels of reflection. The processes that lead to the phenomenon of reflecting about one's thinking and another's thinking are not the same. But improved capacities for self-reflection may result in a more nuanced mind-reading (Dimaggio et al. 2008). Recognizing self-image could be a starter in that process. The core of the self, which is undefined and non-localized,

---

[7] Anosognosia is a condition where there is loss of awareness of a hemiplegia (paralysis on one side of the body).

still requires a via medium for the mind to access, and that cannot be without reflecting upon one's mental states. The core-self is beyond the 'me and the other' divide and hence may not be available as a datum for the phenomenological reflection of the body and the world.

Information is organized through the various self schemas the body and the brain have mapped together. The reorganization of information somehow leads to self-recognition. Recognition involves reflection: Reflecting as to seeing something in an objective manner, and identifying it as either belonging to oneself or not. Through processes of reflection and self-perception, I define my self-concepts, and bring to light personality traits, feelings and behaviours into self-awareness. In spite of self-recognition and self-awareness, at any point I am just *am*. We all are just 'are', just being, at any point, without being aware of a particular object per se. The meta-awareness that does the filtering and integration is connected with the just being, or the core-self.

I think back about past events, think forth about imagined and expected events, and think now on where I am situated. I do not require a mirror-image or a photograph to recognize myself as myself in non-pathological conditions. I recognize the body parts as belonging to me. I recognize the relation between the different body parts, and how that inter-relation is related to my body as a whole. I recognize the body as an integral whole comprising body parts. I recognize that I have a body and I can at times be identified with it as the subject, and at times detach from it as my object of reflection. I recognize the body as a single, indiscrete entity. I also recognize me having, using, and watching the body. Through, and with, the body I recognize the physicality/exteriority of the body and subjectivity/interiority of a deeper reflective consciousness. Thus, the function of reflection is not mere awareness of one's mental states but the provision of a complex, organic relation with the core-self.

6.2.1 Illusion-Based Manipulations of Body-Identification

Yet another experiment that is repeated with variations to question any stable sense of self correlated with body perception and body identification is the 'rubber hand illusion'.[8] A normal subject sits in front of a mirror with his left arm resting on a table in front but concealed from his vision. A dummy rubber left arm is placed on a table directly in front of the subject. While the subject pays attention to the dummy left arm the concealed real left arm and the dummy left arm are touched synchronically with a brush. The subject experienced the tactile sensations caused by the brush to arise from the dummy rubber hand, and also felt that the dummy arm belonged to him. This effect revealed that we distinguish body from other objects and finds it belonging to our self due to certain inter-modal

[8] See Chap. 5.4.

perceptual relations. The integration of certain inter-modal perceptual relations is needed to own the body.

Using a similar illusion that causes inter-sensory bias V. S. Ramachandran got phantom limb patients to view the reflection of their intact arm in a mirror and later the amputated arm appeared to have been resurrected. These illusion-based studies revealed that there is some element in inter-modal sensory correlations that explain the sense of ownership to our body. The sense of ownership to the body at times is described as body image due to 'a stable mental construct of a unitary corporeal self that endures in time' (Ramachandran and Hirstein 1998, p. 1622) which can be 'easily and profoundly modified' (Armel and Ramachandran 2003, p. 1504) it being only a 'transitory internal construct', a 'temporary shell' (p. 1506). It is due to the mental image that 'what is seen' and 'what is felt' are connected.

I wish to raise a phenomenologically fundamental issue that is critical of inter-sensory illusion-based studies. To affirm (a dummy rubber arm as one's) or to deny (a real arm as one's) a prior representation of the body as an integrated entity is essential. Even to disown a limb or neglect a body part as in hemispatial neglect, a prior representation of the body is needed. There needs to be a sense that transfers sensations to other objects, which is continuously present and is not affected by the body-image.

While the body image and the limits of the body-sense can be modified the sense that makes all those decisions, however weird they are, is primary and is the most intact pre-experiential, pre-conceptual core of the self-sense. I think the faulty assumption is in regarding the body-image itself as the self-sense responsible for creating ownership of the body.

What is modified is the neuronal map and not the ability itself to create neuronal maps (such as for the body image). Constantini and Haggard (2007) found that the perception of current sensory stimulation involves assimilation to a 'pre-existing internal representation of the body'. The observational content of my experience is integrated to an already present self-sense that watches and directs the body-sense.

6.2.2 Experience and Ownership

De Vignemonta and Fourneretb (2004) differentiate between the 'minimal self' (Gallagher 2000) and a 'recognitional self' to avoid reducing all of self-recognition to the concept of a self-image. They argue: we have two different kinds of I-thoughts that use different notions of the self. In self-recognition which involves acts like grasping a glass as my own, the sense of agency involves the notion of a 'minimal self' which is instantaneous but carries only a small amount of information about myself that 'I am grasping a glass'. Recognition of one's image in the mirror depends on recognitional criteria that allow me to re-identify myself through time, and hence 'recognitional self' has a richer content and could explain personal identity.

Ownership of a body part, of a relatively simpler act like holding an object, and being the self that owns the body as a whole, are to be distinguished. Though we as humans are good at discrete manipulation of simple acts like picking up something, or exclusively focusing on an object, or single intense feeling, our experiences all the time come with a rich organic complexity.

Hence, experience is not like some archived material, that we can analyse and theorize about its origins and functions in various phases, experience is also not similar to a lab animal that will lie still on the lab table. Experience is best understood in fully lived conditions. We all admit that what give meaning and challenge to our lives is not discrete acts like picking up a glass, or seeing a shade of red color, but the intricately intertwined experiential richness tied to a personal identity.

Most of ownership that we discuss in the context of the body is to explain discrete acts, and is determined by the amount of balance between visual inputs, vestibular mechanisms and proprioception. That the body is owned by me itself is a deeper sensation that ensues from a contiguous and core-self. It is because of a deeper sense of the core-self that changing body maps are translated into meaningful, or strange, experiences and all of them owned by a singular I-am-ness.

In recent times there has been a surge in theories that consider embodied experiences to understand the self and its functions particularly with the help of phenomenology. Subjectivity of the self is attributed to the body itself, and the exteriority of the body to the subject (Zahavi 1999, p. 170). It has been a part of the Western phenomenological tradition to consider the physicality and the subjectivity of the body at the same time. Such a position also warrants attributing singular importance to reflection as an important factor to understand the self-sense.

What is not thought about is that impaired embodiment is hardly needed to understand the curiously phenomenal quality of experience. The uniqueness of my perceptions and my experiences are not only because they are tied to my body but also because they are contained in that part of my self-sense which is directed by subliminal existential features such as my sense of security. How secure, or for that matter, insecure, do I feel? Is my sense of security evident in my actions or is it implicit and gets subtly expressed only through my actions?

6.3 Body and Embodiment

Recent discussions on consciousness, body and embodiment have secured a prominent place with reference to phenomenological traditions. Phenomenological traditions in general and approaches that benefit from these traditions, specifically, consider the body not as a bodily entity but as a subjective phenomenon. The body occupies a centre stage since all activities, cognitive and affective, depend on the body, according to the concept of embodiment.

There is no interaction with the world at large without the intervention of the body. The theory of embodiment extends the physicality of the body to its subjective pervasiveness in all human actions. Essentially, the subjective nature of our perceptions and actions are attributed to the body that encapsulates them. Just as our behaviours are not only an outcome of sensory and motor activities, mental states are not only inner, abstract states. Human actions, intentions and feelings are housed in the body. They are embodied and enacted by being dependent on the body. For this reason, the body is complex and unpredictable. The most fundamental level of embodied agency is that of life itself which brings into focus the philosophy of biology and the theory of the organism (Bruun and Langlais 2003).

To bring in the subjective nature of experiences without the distant ephemerality of the self that carries it has been successfully achieved apropos by the theories that centre on the body. Two central functions are achieved by the focus on body-centrality in analyzing experiences. One, the physicality of the body is softened by the subjectivity of the self; and two, the mysterious, floating locale of the self is grounded on the body.

Discussions that involve studies from neuroscience and neuropsychology shift from an exclusive referral to the brain and consider experience as percolating the whole of human body. A major concept that is used today to understand many bodily functions we perform without conscious effort is 'body representation'. Our ability to receive stimulus through sensations and to respond through motor activities is dependent on a continuously mapped body representation.

> Successful interaction with the environment requires integration of the continuous flow of information that arises from sensory organs, in order to keep track of external stimuli and constantly monitor body status. In addition, interacting within the external world further requires planning, monitoring and executing the appropriate motor acts. Although distinctly processed, sensory information and motor responses are not entirely separable events. Sensory inputs often drive motor behaviour, and planning a movement generates sensory consequences that must be anticipated for actions to be properly carried out. In a cognitive perspective, these processes imply both an immediate elementary analysis of incoming and efferent information, and the possibility of representing inner and outer reality, thus allowing the individual to construct models (or images) of sensations, perceptions and actions (Daprati et al. 2010, p. 756).

The discourse on the brain and the self are today primarily centred on the role and influence of the body and its representation contributing to embodiment of objects, thoughts, actions and feelings. Several features of the experiential self are transferred to the body due to ubiquitous participation of the body in human interactions. The place of the other, other bodies, and the social world, are included in the concept of the self through intersubjectivity.

Subjectivity of the other person is accessible from a second-person perspective (Zahavi 2005, p. 125). The inter-subjective nature of experiences provides an ecological account of human actions. Our actions are contextualized in the past but embedded in the present. For instance, according to Gallaghar, our actions are '… result of a conscious reflection that is embedded or situated in the particular context that is defined by the present circumstance of encountering' (Gallagher 2006, p. 120). Embedded or situated reflection is neither introspective nor focused on body, but is 'a first-person reflective consciousness that is embedded in a pragmatically or socially contextualized situation' (Gallagher and Marcel 1999, p. 25).

How we are perceived by the world, and how we respond to the world around us, are to a great extent guided by the social world and its expectations. There is no experience without the interactive involvement of the other. Our bodily functions such as movement, mental responses such as facial expression, are directed by the inter-subjective world. Phenomenology and phenomenological analysis focus on the world that is disclosed by consciousness. The primary facet of consciousness is that it is intentional and is directed towards 'the other', which is outside. With the claim that phenomenological investigation is prior to the divide between physical exteriority and psychical interiority, Dan Zahavi writes:

> When we investigate appearing objects, we also disclose ourselves as datives of manifestation, as those to whom objects appear. The topic of the phenomenological analyses is consequently not a worldless subject, and phenomenology does not ignore the world in favor of consciousness. On the contrary, phenomenology is interested in consciousness because it is world-disclosing… The phenomenological descriptions take their point of departure in the world we live in. By contrast, to speak of introspection is (tacitly) to endorse the idea that consciousness is inside the head and the world outside. Phenomenology is not concerned with establishing what a given individual might currently be experiencing. Phenomenology is not interested in qualia in the sense of purely individual data that are incorrigible, ineffable, and incomparable. Phenomenology is not interested in psychological processes (in contrast to behavioural processes or physical processes). Phenomenology is interested in the very dimension of givenness or appearance and seeks to explore its essential structures and conditions of possibility. Such an investigation is more fundamental and prior to any divide between psychical interiority and physical exteriority (Zahavi 2011, pp. 17, 18).

But is the phenomenological method foolproof to reveal the inner content of an experience? Are the interpretations of the experience valid at all times? A possible limitation of phenomenology is thus described:

> The problem stems from the dichotomy between inner mind and outer behaviour; the true, inner self is covered by an untrue, outer social world. The phenomenologist acts as archaeologist, digging ever deeper into the inner depths; but the archaeo-phenomenologist can never be sure if the true self has been found, especially because it is the already-buried (false) self which does the digging, using the tools provided by the life world. Because it wants to disinter 'essential meanings', phenomenology fore-closes on an investigation of, not only the opaque-ness of communication or why it is opaque at all, but also the role of communication in the (re)production of the subjective and experiential self in the contextual and material world. Phenomenology has radical intentions, to question the unquestioned, but suggesting a (true) inner world and a (false) outer world denies that there is an internal relationship between them; one merely covers the other, though this cannot be explained (Pile 1993, pp. 124, 125).

6.4 Movement, Agency and Subjectivity

Most of our social interactions, most of the inner-outer transitions, can be brought under the category of movement. The theory of intersubjectivity and its reliance on 'movement' are best illustrated by Jonathan Cole in his narratives of meetings with subjects who are severely challenged in their capacity for locomotion, expression and feeling. The gist of human interactions, which he narrows down to three forms of movement, is designed by the expectations of the society. Hence, beyond bodily disability, it is social disability with which Cole's subjects attempt to cope.

> Almost each and every aspect of our bodily presence is judged by others and so contributes to intersubjectivity. The body in repose, our posture, what we wear and how we groom all add to how others see us and so allow us, to the extent that these can be changed, to position ourselves in relation to others. We also communicate through special movements evolved for intersubjectivity, whether through gesture or voice (language and prosody) or through facial expression. These channels give differing but overlapping information, whether largely factual e.g., some speech, or more emotionally laden e.g., facial expression. Movements may be divided, very simply, into three broad divisions; locomotion, instrumental actions, e.g., dressing, eating, etc., and expressive/emotional/social e.g., some gesture and facial expression.... Subjects who become paralysed as adults, due to spinal cord injury, may lose instrumental action and locomotion while retaining speech and facial expression. In contrast some of those with Möbius Syndrome, the congenital absence of facial expression, may have profound problems in emotional expression with near normal instrumental and locomotion action (Cole 2009, p. 344).

Visual feedback with inputs from other sensory modalities, coupled with proprioceptive capabilities, accounts for our ease in movement and motor activities. It is not an exaggeration to say that movement is the hallmark of body as a physical entity which connects with subjective qualities. Perhaps this is the reason investigators like Cole equate movement as a function that interstice between motor activities and emotional expressions. The range of the body and its movement is extended from motor responses to nuanced gestural and facial expressions.

Will the posturing of movement as a subjective and social function impede with the physical distinction of the body and the self, and, more importantly, the conceptual distinction of the first person and the third person accounts? Such a problematic is envisaged by some of the phenomenological considerations of body and movement. For instance, a study that is conducted on 'body experts', a group of ballet dancers, reveals intriguing ideas on self-perception and agency, based on the argument that subjectivity and intersubjectivity ought not to be equated. The authors write:

> ... [I]t is problematic that phenomenological investigations of the body (e.g., Merleau-Ponty 1964; Gallagher 2005) primarily focus either on pathological movements disrupted in their adaptation to the task or environment or disrupted in their fluidity or on very simple and rather isolated everyday movements like holding a cup or pointing to one's nose. Such movements neglect important components of acceleration and deceleration or the effects of gravity, which are evidently present in whole-body movements (Legrand and Ravn 2009, p. 393).
>
> ... [Á]ny 'I move' never occurs in a vacuum but as part of a physical context. Moving and experiencing ones body cannot be reduced to the experiential processing of information about the body itself but rather encompass the experiential processing of information which merely concern the body indirectly while being centred on the exteroceptive perception of non-bodily elements of the world (Legrand and Ravn 2009, p. 400)

Without equating subjectivity and intersubjectivity, first-person and second-person perspectives, this study presents a fresh approach to agency as constitutive not just of agent's authorship and but also of the experiencer's visual ability to control and access body movements, receive sensory information from one's and another's body to control movement, and to base movement upon imagination and transformativity (Legrand and Ravn 2009, pp. 389–408). Agency is defined as the sense of authorship of one's actions (Kircher and Leube 2003). It is described as the 'Who System', with underlying cognitive processes (Georgieff and Jeannerod 1998). Owing to the excess of first-person content in experience, the essential expressions of 'raw feelings', called 'primary self-experiences' in cognitive sciences, are not included in the conceptualization of agency. This is one reason that much of the discussion on agency in the context of consciousness and action is limited to sensory-motor activities and impairments.

Of course, the question that stays back is whether human agency is just a product of intentions and physiological capabilities. Finally, is not human agency dependent on the capabilities of the person to engage in an act and fulfil it as a whole person involving his or her being as a whole? Agency will be an important concept in the coming years to explore the nature of consciousness and also to understand how much subjectivity can be extracted from consciousness and how much objectivity can be attributed to it. A major problem for working on pure objectivity of consciousness is the fact that at any given moment to observe the observation of observation will not be possible since all the three acts cannot be brought at one point of time.

To conceptualize agency from a positive framework of the possibility of experiences, the methodology will have to accommodate both the third-person content of experience and the first-person agency of consciousness. Such a method might first help to analyse and then resolve various phases of agency into a level that might be depicted as acausal and apodeictic. This would demand considering agency not as a pole but more a field through which all experiences pass (Kircher and Leube 2003). We need to look at how first-person experiences and accounts could be made a component in third-person approaches.

The cognitive and neural aspects of agency and the primary sense of self are inextricably intertwined in an individual's experience. Our experience tells us that to have an experience and derive meaning from it, both authorship and a sense of self are required. Experience is made meaningful by the continued 'feeling' of the self. A sense of enduring and pervasive identity is the starting point of all experiences. The story as well as the narrative modes of conscious experience (Petranker 2003) might help us to balance between the fringes of pure subjectivity and pure objectivity of consciousness. With a third-person approach we can capture only the discrete frames of the vent part by part. But the challenge is that the content of consciousness undergoes a series of changes such that each frame or part gets redefined and reconstituted in the act of 'capture'. Since observation per se needs another observation to be an object of inquiry, at any given time a subjective component persists impervious to the act of observation.

The knower is not just intricately but indivisibly connected with observation due to which we can know only the contents of observation and not the observer per se. According to Vedantic epistemology, consciousness by itself never becomes the knower, the act of knowing and the known. Consciousness sustains the triad of objective discreteness without being a part of the triad.

6.5 Core-Self and Self Correlates

Seeing oneself and seeing the other are two different domains as far as recognition is concerned, though they are available to us in an entwined manner. Francisco Varela, who initiated the introduction of phenomenology in the cognitive sciences, commenced from the premise, inspired by Merleau-Ponty, that bodies are to be seen as both physical structures and as lived, experiential structures, as both outer and inner, biological and phenomenological (Varela et al. 1991). By its constitution the lived body is both physical and subjective. This contention presents the philosophically poignant but problematic position that one's body does not become an object like any other object when perceived. On the other hand, the body becomes subjective by being perceived. The perceivability of the body makes it subjective.

The body-centredness immanent in the view—though it benefits science and brings to the forefront an elevated nature of the body and relegated status of the self—extols the body as the be all and end all of life. Varela[9] and others, inspired by the Buddhist tradition of Nagarjuna (second century CE), which upholds a middle path of no-self theory, and supported by the non-physical attributes of body as discussed by Merleau-Ponty, have heralded the mainstream scenario in today's neuropsychology which extends the bounds of body to the self. Varela writes:

> … emphasis on mutual specification that enables us to negotiate a middle path between the Scylla of cognition as the recovery of a pregiven outer world (realism) and the Charybdis of cognition as the projection of a pregiven inner world (idealism). These two extremes both take representation as their central notion: in the first case representation is used to recover what is outer; in the second case it is used to project what is inner. Our intention is to bypass entirely this logical geography of inner versus outer by studying cognition not as recovery or projection but as embodied action (Varela et al. 1991, p. 172).

The inextricable connection between the human spirit and the physical body is once again brought to our attention, reminding us alternate ontologies of the body and the self in other traditions such as Advaita Vedanta. It is due to want of in-between concepts to bridge the highly subjective self and the perceptually physical body that the classically believed functions of the experiencer-self are given to the body.[10] This for sure has enlivened a body which otherwise would have faced death because of its sheer physicality.

---

[9] '… in the logic of Darwin's account of evolution and the Buddhist analysis of experience into co-dependent arising, we are concerned with the processual transformation of the past into the future through the intermediary of transitional forms that in themselves have no permanent substance' (Varela et al. 1991, p. 116).

[10] In Advaita, the closest concept that comes to a lived phenomenological body is '*jiva*' which is defined as that which is limited by its physical, subtle and causal bodies'. *Jiva* is a doer and enjoyer of its actions, makes its intentions and harbours memories. *Jiva* is the twilight space of the physical body and the subjective experiencer. Self, which is *atman*, is beyond *Jiva* and remains pure consciousness.

The danger and the problematic in this trend is that by housing the functions of an unperceived self in the perceived body the scope of the core-self is limited and foreclosed. Transformations of the self become transformations of the lived body. The idea of the core-self that is unperceived yet present deepens the body-sense by placing it within a deeper self-sense. The lived body, contrary to the phenomenological position, becomes an object for the core-self.

Let us come back to some of the questions this discussion commenced with. Can the phenomenal and ontological aspects of the self treated identically or even interchangeably? The lived body and the bodily-self presented in the 'clinical tales' are narratives of the fragile self defined by the social other and the physical body. The self presented in much of neuropsychiatry is a spliced and mixed up hybrid of the shifting attributes of a social self and an unperceived non-physical self. Does the phenomenological attributes of the neuropsychiatric self blur the fundamental debate between the spiritual and physical nature of the self? Is the classic body-mind debate now receding and giving room for brain-self debate, but in the process eliminating the core attributes of a non-physical self?

The essential 'function' of the self is to make 'sense' of information received electrochemically, and from multiple sense-organs (including mind). What is it to make sense? What is it to have motivation, intention, the sense of free will, meaning and purpose? Are these the inhabitants of a phenomenal body or of the core-self that could be described as unperceived pure consciousness?

One of the major puzzles that brain scientists face is the curious play that the brain engages with the self and brain's tremendous capacity for regeneration and remapping. There is something that 'tells' the brain to change according to altering conditions. The brain seems to be a continuously adapting mechanism, based on the cues it receives from what I would call 'self-correlates' of consciousness, such as love, hope, affective engagement, compassion, happiness, creativity, and other such positive qualities.

However much we reduce the human self and identity to neural processes, there seems to remain an irreducible, inseparable, core-self that helps the experiencer self marked by human sensitivities and frailties. These are not just neural functions but signposts that the self creates. The self-sense through some mechanism unknown to us, has the capacity to overpower the neural limits and act on its own, because at times we are able to defy physical conditions and express without a physical medium. In an article entitled 'The Power of Hope', M. Scott Haig writes about his patient with brain tumour who made a spectacular comeback from coma, though for a few moments, to say 'goodbye' to his family.

> David's head was literally stuffed with lung cancer. I was called into take care of his hip and pelvic bones broken by the growing metastases. ...The cerebral machine that talked and wondered, winked and sang, the machine that remembered jokes and birthdays and where the big fish hid on hot days, was nearly gone, replaced by lumps of haphazardly growing gray stuff. Gone with that machine seemed David as well. No expression, no response to anything we did to him. As far as I could tell, he was just not there... Saturday morning the sun poured in as I checked the room. The bed was at chest height, made up and empty, with clean, fresh sheets over the vinyl mattress. As I turned to leave, I was blocked by a nurse, an older Irish lady with a doleful look on her face. She had taken care of David last night. 'He

> woke up, you know, doctor—just after you left—and said goodbye to them all. Like I'm talking to you right here. Like a miracle. He talked to them and patted them and smiled for about five minutes. Then he went out again, and he passed in the hour.
>
> ... But it wasn't David's brain that woke him up to say goodbye that Friday. His brain had already been destroyed. ...It's wonderful to see, such tangible evidence of that fine thing's power over the mere clumps of particles that, however pretty, will eventually clump differently and vanish (Scott Haig 2007).

Several neuropsychiatrists today use the first-person account of experiences of their patients to understand the construal of agency and experience in challenging situations. These accounts have brought in the humanizing picture of the brain presenting an alternate perspective to understand the brain and the body. Jonathan Cole in his classic books narrates the experiences and responses of patients with spinal cord injury and Mobius syndrome[11] that result in movement disability and emotional impoverishment. He narrates the unusual condition of patients who have extreme difficulty with movement due to the lack of the senses of touch and proprioception below the neck. Cole's narratives explain how they experience and project their agency (Cole 1998, 2004, 2009),[12] and how embodiment matters for some and not for others.

> ... [A] young student with bilateral facial palsy (due to a medical condition, sarcoid) was robbed of facial expression whilst at college. Though outwardly confident and brash, he was essentially shy. During the weeks and months without facial movement he found it crucial to express himself with a clarity, in speech and gesture, he had not previously contemplated. He dropped out of his course for a year. On his return, and looking back, he suggested that his time out had been a good thing. He had been forced to mature, to think about things in new and deeper ways, allowing him improved confidence. His immobile face had been a shield and protector rather than a prison (Cole 2009, p. 349).

In *Still Lives*, Cole (2004) gives an account of the responses he received from people with quadriplegia due to spinal cord injuries for the question, 'What it is like to live without sensation and movement in the body?' If the body is dysfunctional, where does the self reside? Cole finds that there is no single or simple answer. Cole narrates the stories of quadriplegic patients in wheel chair, with the help of six expressions that can only be explained relating them to the core-self. Studying their experiences Cole titles the chapters of the book with expressions of self-correlates: 'enduring', 'exploring', 'experimenting', 'observing', 'empowering', and 'continuing'.

To quote from some of the narratives:

> IW suffers from an acute sensory neuropathy in which large fibers below the neck have been destroyed by illness. As a result IW has no proprioceptive function and no sense of touch below the neck. At the onset of the neuropathy IW's initial experience was of complete loss of control of posture and movement. He could not sit up or move his limbs in any controllable way. Maintaining posture is, for him, an activity rather than an automatic

[11] Mobius syndrome is a neurological disorder characterized by facial paralysis.

[12] Books by Jonathan Cole, such as *About Face* (1998) and *Still Lives* (2004) look at the social and personal difficulties faced by patients with unusual experiences and how they manage to reconcile and make progress with the help of 'sheer effort, will power and an ingenious collection of motor tricks'. Also, read Gallagher's (2004) interview with Cole.

> process. His movement requires constant visual and mental concentration. In darkness he is unable to control movement; when he walks he cannot daydream, but must concentrate constantly on his movement. When he writes he has to concentrate on holding the pen and on his body posture.
>
> For the first three months, even with a visual perception of the location of his limbs, he could not control his movement. In the course of the following two years, while in a rehabilitation hospital, he gained sufficient motor control to feed himself, write, and walk. He went on to master everyday motor tasks of personal care, housekeeping, and those movements required to work in an office setting (Gallagher and Cole 1995, p. 371).

Cole quotes from the narrative of one of his young subjects:

> ... I never burst into tears because, from the early stages of living with the injury, I have seen the whole thing as a challenge. How do I overcome so and so? How do I deal with this? How do I come to terms with that? I never thought, 'I can't do that' (Cole 2004, p. 49, quoted in Cole 2009, p. 347).

These accounts tell us how the hope for betterment and the extra positive effort, in spite of the neural challenge, makes the self-sense stable and help overpower its own slippery and shifting features.[13] The self is studied through an engaged self-exploratory method with the intervention of values and positive dispositions. What is significant about such neuropsychiatric literature is the shift in focus from the third-person neural data to the first-person qualities of will power and self-effort. The first-person qualities are being recognized as pertinent to cope up with challenging physical conditions and to help achieve some neural and experiential progress.

Is the pursuit for flourishing deeply engraved in the humans? The published narratives from Cole and the several unpublished narratives that we are familiar with in the lives of our friends and acquaintances tell us that deep down somewhere our spirit guides our fragile body-sense and the self-sense that holds it to respond to challenges so as to optimize wellbeing. Our ability to draw energy and courage to face physical disabilities, mental challenges and emotional conflicts indicates a core-self that is undefined and not reducible to the self-sense that upholds the bodily-self. Core-self is the adherent base of all subjective experiences, that shines up our discrete states of mind and body, giving immediate knowledge and awareness.

Detached and 'disembodied', reductionist theories of the self do not give the space for exploring its own possibilities. In Damasio's hopeful words: 'Nature lacks a plan for human flourishing, but nature's humans are allowed to devise such a plan' (2003, p. 287).

[13] According to the *Bhagavad Gita*, it is by individual effort alone that one can rise above oneself—'uplift yourself by your own efforts' (*Bhagavad Gita* 6:5).

6.6 Brain–Self Connectors

We might argue qualitative awareness to be either an emergent phenomenon, or not, of neural firings. Such awareness percolates into the self-sense in myriad forms known only to the experiencer—twitch, pain, tickle etc. all tailor-made for that person and his or her experience. There is an awareness that gives the grand sense that 'this body and mind belongs to me'. Even when a body part is disowned or unrecognized, there is a feeling of the body and the self in a tight knit. Whatever is available to the body-sense and the self-sense at any point is put together and a reference generated through the self that 'it is me'.

The core-self can be defined as the substratum, of pure consciousness, and the beholder and referent point of all sensations, feelings, thoughts, intentions, desires, actions and the sense of security. The core-self is the very core of being from where everything else, the body and the other, me and the world, seems to rise, reside and disappear. However much we subjectivize the body and the body-sense, these cannot become the core-self.

If we consider the body-sense and the self-sense as layers not laid on one another but moving in concentric fashion, then we can also understand why their functions defy theories of mutual reduction: Why subjectivity is overridden by the physicality of experience, and why brain functions are overridden by the subjective quality of neural firings.

The brain and the self-sense are connected not just at the level of the body and cognitive functions but also at the levels of unique human capabilities of freedom, choice-making and taking responsibility. Even though our decision-making processes are determined by unconscious processing, our experience entails not just motor activity or sensory response but a sense of freedom in expressing and beholding such responses as a part of our personhood. We are free not just in moving our limbs, perceiving or lifting objects, but in integrating those actions and perceptions into a plenum of reflective and introspective system. Free will in this sense is the subtle quality of the core-self and not just a philosophical idea that can be tossed around by polemists. The reflective and introspective processes that we possess organically are not free *from* something, but are essentially free. The brain and the self-sense are connected in the ontological space of essential freedom.

References

Armel, K. C., & Ramachandran, V. S. (2003). Projecting sensations to external objects: evidence from skin conductance response. *Proceedings of the Royal Society of London: Biological, 270*, 1499–1506.

Bitbol, M., & Petitmengin, C. (2011). On pure reflection: A reply to Dan Zahavi. *Journal of Consciousness Studies, 18*(2), 24–37.

Bruun, H., & Langlais, R. (2003). On the embodied nature of action. *Acta Sociologica, 46*(1), 31–49.

Cole, J. (1998). *About Face*. Cambridge, MA: The MIT Press.

Cole, J. (2004). *Still lives: Narratives of spinal cord injury*. Boston, MA: MIT Press.

Cole, J. (2009). Impaired embodiment and intersubjectivity. *Phenomenology and the Cognitive Sciences, 8*(3), 343–360.

Costantini, M., & Haggard, P. (2007). The rubber hand illusion: Sensitivity and reference frame for body ownership. *Consciousness and Cognition, 16*, 229–240.

Cytowic, R. (2002). *Synesthesia: A union of the senses*. Cambridge: Bradford.

Damasio, A. (1999). *Feeling of what happens: Body and emotion in the making of consciousness*. London: Heinemann.

Damasio, A. (2003). *Looking for spinoza: Joy, sorrow and the feeling brain*. London: William Heinemann.

Daprati, E., Sirigu, A., & Nico, D. (2010). Body and movement: Consciousness in the parietal lobes. *Neuropsychologia, 48*, 756–762.

Dimaggio, G., Lysaker, P., Carcione, A., Nicolo, G., & Semerari, A. (2008). Know yourself and you shall know the other… to a certain extent: Multiple paths of influence of self-reflection on mindreading. *Consciousness and Cognition, 17*, 778–789.

Feinberg, T. E. (2001). *Altered egos: How the brain creates the self*. New York: Oxford University Press.

Gallagher, S. (2000). Philosophical conceptions of the self: Implications for cognitive science. *Trends in the Cognitive Sciences, 4*(1), 14–21.

Gallagher, S. (2004). Nailing the lie: An interview with Jonathan Cole. *In Journal of Consciousness Studies, 11*(2), 3–22.

Gallagher, S. (2005). *How the body shapes the mind*. Oxford: Oxford University Press.

Gallagher, S. (2006). Where's the action? Epiphenomenalism and the problem of free will. In W. Banks, S. Pockett, & S. Gallagher (Eds.), *Does consciousness cause behaviour: An investigation of the nature of volition* (pp. 109–124). Cambridge: MIT Press.

Gallagher, S., & Cole, J. (1995). Body schema and body image in a deafferented subject. *Journal of Mind and Behavior, 16*, 369–390.

Gallagher, S., & Marcel, A. (1999). The self in contextualized action. *Journal of Consciousness Studies, 6*(4), 4–30.

Gallup, G. G. (1977). Self recognition in primates: A comparative approach to the bidirectional properties of consciousness. *American Psychologist, 32*(5), 329–338.

Georgieff, N., & Jeannerod, M. (1998). Beyond consciousness of external reality: A "Who" system for consciousness of action and self-consciousness. *Consciousness and Cognition, 7*, 465–477.

Heilman, K. M., Barrett, A. M., & Adair, J. C. (1998). Possible mechanisms of anosognosia: A defect in self-awareness. *Philosophical Transactions: Biological Sciences, 353*(1377), 1903–1909.

Kircher, T. T., & Leube, D. T. (2003). Self-consciousness, self-agency and schizophrenia. *Consciousness and Cognition, 12*(4), 656–669.

Legrand, D., & Ravn, S. (2009). Perceiving subjectivity in bodily movement: The case of dancers. *Phenomenology and the Cognitive Sciences, 8*, 389–408.

Merleau-Ponty, M. (1964). *The Primacy of Perception*. Evanston, IL: Northwestern University Press.

Sastri, & Nagaraja Rao, G. (1990). *Natya Sastra Samgraha* (3rd ed.,Vol. 1).Tanjavaur: Saraswati Mahal Library.

Petranker, J. (2003). Inhabiting conscious experience: Engaged objectivity in the first-person study of consciousness. *Journal of Consciousness Studies, 10*(12), 3–23.

Philippi, C. L., & Feinstein, J. (2012). Preserved self-awareness following extensive bilateral brain damage to the Insula, Anterior Cingulate, and Medial Prefrontal Cortices. *PLoS ONE, 7*(8), e38413.

Pile, S. (1993). Human agency and human geography revisited: A critique of 'New Models' of the self. *Transactions of the Institute of British Geographers, 18*(1), 122–139.

Ramachandran, V. S. (2003). *The emerging mind*. London: The BBC in association with Profile Books Ltd.

Ramachandran, V. S., & Blakeslee, S. (1998). *Phantoms in the brain*. New York: William Morrow.
Ramachandran, V. S., & Hirstein, W. (1998). The perception of phantom limbs: The D. O. Hebb lecture. *Brain, 121*(1), 1603–1630.
Sacks, O. (1985). *The man who mistook his wife for a hat and other clinical tales*. New York: Summit Books.
Scott Haig, M. (2007, January). The brain: The power of hope. *Time*, 58–59.
Varela, F., Thompson, E., & Rosch, E. (1991). *The embodied mind: cognitive science and human experience*. Cambridge, MA: MIT Press.
Vignemonta, Fd, & Fourneretb, P. (2004). The sense of agency: A philosophical and empirical review of the "Who" system. *Consciousness and Cognition, 13*, 1–19.
Zahavi, D. (1999). *Self-awareness and alterity: A phenomenological investigation*. Evanston: Northwestern University Press.
Zahavi, D. (2005). *Self and subjectivity: Investigating the first-person perspective*. Cambridge, MA: MIT Press.
Zahavi, D. (2011). Varieties of reflection. *Journal of Consciousness Studies, 18*(2), 9–19.

Chapter 7
The Feel Factor: Qualia and the Affective Markers of Experience

What is it that makes us human? It's not something you can program. You can't put it into a chip. It's the strength of the human heart. The difference between us and the machines.

—From 'Terminator Salvation'
As Marcus gives his heart to John Connor

It is commonly agreed that all our experiences come with a subjective quality which provokes, invokes and enriches its contents. What we identify as 'my own self', 'me', and 'mine', is felt by us and expressed for others through our emotions. It is the feel factor of emotions that is recognized and gauged by others through our facial expressions, tone of voice, innuendos in speaking, and the general disposition of the body.

Emotions are variously interpreted as: physiological changes caused so as to produce appropriate behavioural responses; aesthetic agents that invoke relish in one who enjoys a piece of art; tools of communication that tell another person about the warmth or coldness of one's personality; markers of attitude for inter-subjective transference; valence of one's perception about life and life goals. Emotions carve our personal identities, without which others will find it hard to understand us and communicate with us. They are the narrators of physical, mental and social health for ourselves and for others. Through our emotions we know how much we are in 'control' and how much we are involved. While from one point of view they guide neural mechanisms for physiological and chemical balance, on the other emotions enhance self-expression and the presentation of the person.

The history of interest in studying emotions is as old as ancient Egyptian and Ayurvedic medicine. Several questions persisted since then continue to inspire the study of emotions and bring in the role of the brain, the body, and the self, interspersed by the influence of environment, society, art, and one's character. How and why does brain activity generate emotions? Or does it? Are emotions evolutionary vestiges or enhancers of experience? Are feelings and emotions different, and have different roles to play? Are there feelings that are not necessarily dependent on sensations? Can we have perceptions without feelings? Are feelings emergent

S. Menon, *Brain, Self and Consciousness*, Studies in Neuroscience, Consciousness and Spirituality, DOI: 10.1007/978-81-322-1581-3_7,

properties of experience or are they discrete cognitive events? Can emotions be understood within the framework of neuroscience?

How do emotions reason and respond? What are the rational and cognitive components in emotions? Or, in other words, what is 'known' through emotions? Can we think exclusively as a rational entity, or is it that our emotions influence the arguments that we form using rational activities in advance? What is the relation between emotion and memory? What is the role of emotion in autistic subjects? How is social behaviour guided by our emotional responses? What is it to sense sensation, and sense feeling? How are physical sensations and mental feels presented in a united manner to the subjective experience? Can we discount the belongingness and owning features of feelings, and how adequate are the concepts of qualia and representationalism to represent these subjective nuances? What is the role of bodily subjectivity in framing a continuum of self-experience?

Yet another contention about feelings is that they are not necessarily dependent on sensations, and that there is the possibility of perceptions without feelings. Or, in other words, what is it to sense sensation, and sense feeling? Is there a difference between these two kinds of senses that we possess? And if they are different, how are physical sensations and mental feels presented in a united manner to our subjective experiences?

In spite of these enchanting questions that lure human imagination, emotions give us a sense of belongingness and owning through our feelings. They are the spokespersons of our inner life and aid in framing a continuum of self-experience and social interactions. We feel the other through our emotions. The other gets to know us through the expressions of our emotions.

7.1 The Feel Factor

At any given time, a subject has multiplicity of experiences (Bayne and Chalmers 2003). These experiences are distinct from each other. At the same time, they are unified by being aspects of a single encompassing state of consciousness. This total state is not a conjunction of different conscious states. But it is another conscious state in its own right.

Experiences come to us as a unified whole. There is a fundamental and intrinsic unity to all experiences. The unity is experienced primarily through and by the subject of experience. Hence, we also know that we do not have just one single unified sensory experience but multi-sensorial experiences. We receive five sensory experiences that are directed to one object or several objects at the same time. I could be eating an apple, watching the blue waves, feeling the breeze on my skin, smelling the fresh air, hearing the distant call of the boatman—all these are experienced at the same time with clear distinctive feels for each. At the same time, I could be also revelling in what could be described as a nostalgic feeling about the rivers in Kerala.

All these feelings are experienced in a discrete as well as wholesome manner. Each discrete sensory experience is presented to us as a unified whole. At the same time, multi-sensorial experiences are together presented to us as a unified whole. Our experience presents all of its different content in one unitary beholdence. They all are cohered in a unitary subject, which is my-self.

7.1.1 Representationalism

In order to commence a discussion on emotion, it is important to understand the class of concepts to which it might belong. All components that produce or contribute to the subjective nature of experience, including our feelings, belong to the class of qualia. Emotions and such other entities are perhaps even responsible for generating the qualia of experience.

A strong assumption among the philosophers of mind is that all mental facts and states can be explained in terms of natural science. Mind can be naturalized and explained reductively in terms of neural functions. Emotions are also of natural kinds that can be known objectively and are marked biologically. Is this true? Have we even succeeded in defining emotion without much vagueness?

> … I suggest that progress in the scientific understanding of emotion is not, as one might assume, hampered by disagreements. Instead, I argue that progress is limited by the wide acceptance of assumptions that are not warranted by the available empirical evidence. These assumptions can be summarized by one core idea: Certain emotions (at least those referred to in Western cultures by the words 'anger,' 'sadness,' 'fear,' 'disgust,' and 'happiness') are given to us by nature. That is, they are natural kinds, or phenomena that exist independent of our perception of them. Each emotion is thought to produce coordinated changes in sensory, perceptual, motor, and physiological functions that, when measured, provide evidence of that emotion's existence. The natural-kind view of emotion has been productive in defining the boundaries for the scientific study of emotion and continues to guide scientific discourse: It underlies the major questions, the experimental designs, and the interpretation of empirical findings that characterize emotion research as a domain of scientific inquiry. In the pages that follow, however, I suggest that the natural-kind view of emotion may be the result of an error of arbitrary aggregation … our perceptual processes lead us to aggregate emotional processing into categories that do not necessarily reveal the causal structure of the emotional processing. I suggest that, as a result, the natural-kind view has outlived its scientific value and now presents a major obstacle to understanding what emotions are and how they work (Barrett 2006a, p. 29).

Another view that argues against the naturalist supposition of emotion holds that the subjective nature of experience cannot be naturalized since the processes responsible are rooted in representational structures of mind. Amongst philosophers of mind the notion of 'mental representation' is a major contender to describe qualia in terms of cognition. Primarily, mental representation is a concept that has arisen from the theories of cognitive science.

Computational psychology and cognitive neurosciences postulate different structures and processes towards describing representation. These structures are rarely parts of common experience, but often linguistic concepts for representing the phenomenal and the feel factor of experience. Computational theory of mind suggests that brain is like a computer and mental processes are computations. Metzinger cautions such approaches:

> … Because many such philosophers are superb at analyzing the deeper structure of language, they often fall into the trap of analyzing the conscious mind as if it were *itself* a linguistic entity, based not on dynamical self-organization in the human brain, but on a disembodied system of rule-based information processing (Metzinger 2003, p. 4).

From classic times the mind has been viewed as consisting of cognition, affect (emotion) and conation (motivation). A valid criticism against the approaches in cognitive sciences is that though the claim is that it is the 'mind' which is studied, only one aspect of the mind is projected to represent the whole of mind, namely cognition. Emotion and motivation are as important, or at times more important than the cognitive rules we apply in life. And therefore our acts are not just 'lifting objects' or 'standing up' and 'using linguistic rules'. Ledoux (2002) makes the following perceptive argument:

> The fact that emotion and motivation are not studied by cognitive science makes sense if cognitive science is regarded as a science of cognition, but is troubling if the field is supposed to be the science of mind. A mind without feelings and strivings (the kind of mind traditionally studied in cognitive science) might be able to solve certain problems given by a cognitive psychologist, but it doesn't stack up well as the mental foundation of a self. The kind of mind modeled by cognitive science can, for example, play chess very well, and can even be programmed to cheat. But it is not plagued with guilt when it cheats, or distracted by love, anger, or fear. Neither is it self-motivated by a competitive streak, or by envy or compassion. If we are to understand how the mind, through the brain, makes us who we are, we need to consider the *whole* mind, not just the parts that subserve thinking (LeDoux 2002, p. 14).

The growing interest in 'affective neuroscience' as demonstrated primarily by the works of Panksepp argues that if the focus in understanding consciousness is shifted to the realm of emotions, better results might emerge.

> …many of the scientific dilemmas of the twentieth century, including the Computational Theory of Mind advocated by many cognitive scientists, were created by situating all of consciousness (i.e. the capacity of have 'awareness' of experiences) just at the very top of the brain, especially the sensory-perceptual and ecutive regions of the brain. The instinctual-emotional action apparatus, the source of raw emotional experiences, that helps weave together a foundational form of organismic coherence (perhaps a core-SELF) was provided no role in consciousness. That view prevailed, and was well-tolerated, in preference to the ever increasing empirical evidence during the second half of the twentieth century that affective consciousness perhaps the primal form of 'core consciousness'—had evolutionarily ripened into experiential states within the ancient subcortical brain networks. These foundational basic emotional and motivational urges of all mammals, which monitor vital life qualities, are the foundation of mind (Panksepp et al. 2012, p. 15).

An offshoot of the attempt to focus on a limited context of experience is to learn the behaviour of single neurons and identify them with exclusive cognitive functions. A report, quoting the findings announced at an annual meeting of the Society for Neuroscience, claims that scientists who examine single neurons in the human brain have successfully identified individual brain cells responding to particular stimuli such as pictures of individual people and objects.[1] They have also found that people can control the firing of single neurons. These research findings may help scientists understand the cognitive processes and how individual brain cells respond to particular stimuli. The hope from such studies is that the findings may find application in building machines that can be controlled by human thoughts. Such machines could help people who cannot move like those who suffer from quadriplegia.

Is there a potential danger lingering in such exclusivist studies that conceive human experience and action discretely, and out of context? The field of single neuron studies throws open a highly controversial subject as far as human ethics is concerned. The possibility of knowing how a single neuron stores information also suggests ways for manipulating it for pedagogic and medical reasons. Such a possibility questions the role and place of the human self, agency and free will.

7.1.2 Bodily Subjectivity and its Qualities

The place of the self in dominant philosophical theories of brain-mind relation is understood to a great extent by reviewing how representationalism conceptualizes qualia, the essential subjective nature of experience that possesses feeling. Philosophers who hold a strong representationalist view defines the phenomenal (experiential) character of an experience as one and the same as its poised, abstract, non-conceptual, intentional content (Tye 1995, p. 176). The phenomenal aspects of an experience in not present in the neural events or in an unified experience. They present themselves at the closure of the experience. Phenomenal unity comes along with the closure of experience under conjunction (Tye 1995, p. 84). Just as meaning of a word is not quality of the word the phenomenal character of an experience is not a quality experience possesses (Tye, 1997). The content of qualia is non-conceptual and is not neurophysiological, according to this emergent theory. There are also views that contest the view that emotions have definable boundaries in the brain or the body (Barrett 2006a).

We have varied feelings for different shades of the colour red. Even if we do not have different concepts for those shades of red, we are capable of many more feelings than concepts. Feelings lie in the interface of conceptual and non-conceptual domains. They are the output of the early, largely modular, sensory processing and are the input to another system of higher-level cognitive processing. Differing from Fodor, Tye holds that a sentence is not enough to represent a sensation, as a sensation includes some kind of 'mapping' of the domain to which it refers. For example, pain is about the body, and needs a way to represent the body parts that are affected by pain. Sentences lack this map-like representational power. Tye proposes an 'encompassing experience' (he questions it and dismisses it subsequently

[1] See PHYSORG.com; http://www.physorg.com/news175417796.html; accessed on 8 June 2011.

since it leads to infinite regress) that includes all other experiences within itself. Experience is the bearer of the unified phenomenology (Tye 2003, p. 20).

The question of unity of experience is crucial in understanding the feel factor in an experience. Does each sensory experience come with a feel unique to it? Or is there is only a single experience with a rich feel? How are the distinct feels of discrete sensory experiences retained in a single, unified experience?

Feinberg writes:

> When the neurologist observes the brain experiencing 'pain' from the outside, she sees specific patterns of neural activity that can be accurately defined, but cannot see in the brain something neurological that is equivalent to the experience of 'pain.' When viewed from the outside therefore, the quale 'pain' really does not exist materially. From the outside point of view, my patient's qualia are illusory. Qualia are personal and the relationship between a given brain and a given mind differs whether one is the person having that brain and that experience (Feinberg 2001, p. 147).

Tye dismisses the very possibility of a metalevel of unification of sensory experiences. His key argument is that unification happens at the end of the experience and is part of the processes of representation.

> … to the question of what unifies different simultaneous bodily experiences is that it is a pseudoquestion, based on a mistaken assumption. There is only a single bodily experience at a time, an experience with a very rich and complex bodily phenomenal content. Qualities that are experienced in undergoing bodily experience—qualities that are *not* qualities of experiences but rather qualities of bodily disturbances, if they are qualities of anything—are experienced together at a time by entering into this *shared* content. In this way, the painfulness of a pain, the itchiness of an itch, the ticklishness of a tickle are phenomenologically unified (Tye 2003, p. 66).

7.2 Qualia and Non-physical Feelings

Can we have a feel without a sense-experience? How do we understand the mental feels we have that are not necessarily dependent on sensations?

Much of the discussion on qualia is dependent on the body and the examples are centred on bodily subjectivity. We know that we can have a 'feel' without physical objects invoked by our thoughts, fears, elations, and such mental phenomena. At certain occasions, the 'feel' extends from the mind to the spirit through the values we cherish, such as altruism and compassion.

Tye's view on qualia as a representation brings in the body as the centre of subjectivity and thus discourages the scope for a non-physical, non-embodied self. He argues that feelings are not properties of experience, and that it is the bodily subjectivity which plays the role of a continuing self. Tye favours an intentional account of consciousness. But, in actual experience, we could argue that there is a greater role played by non-intentional consciousness, a consciousness that is not directed towards any object.

The feel-experience that is directed from an object presupposes a non-intentional, pure, core-self ('introspective consciousness' as termed by Tye) until that experience happens. Also, the core-self stays in a different form in the background, so to say, as the reflective awareness (not the 'responsive consciousness' suggested by Tye). It is the reflective awareness that enables the phenomenal character of the experience to be related to the subject. We are able to reflect upon the feel factor because of the non-intentional consciousness that presents itself continuously, without a break.

Every experience, along with the distinct sensory feel, comes with another awareness which is of a 'belongingness' or 'owning', as Kant says. But the ownership itself is an expression of the non-intentional consciousness. The Eastern tradition of Vedanta describes this as one of the characteristics of the ontological self which serves as the adhering entity, enabling us to aware sensory experience(s).

The strong representationalism defended by Dretske (1995), Tye (1995), Lycan (1995) and others holds that the feel is a representation of a certain kind which can be specified in functionalist or other physicalist terms. There is no need for recourse to properties of any ontologically 'new' sort (Tye 1995). According to Lycan:

> [we can never]... specify what it is about the brain that is responsible for consciousness, but I am sure that whatever it is not inherently miraculous. The problem arises, I want to suggest, because we are cut off by our very cognitive constitution from achieving a conception of that natural property of the brain (or of consciousness) that accounts for the psychophysical link (Lycan 1996, p. 160).

There is no continuing self, and 'no such things as selves exist in the world. Nobody ever *was* or *had* a self. All that ever existed were conscious self-models that could not be recognized *as* models' (Metzinger 2003, p. 1). 'Also, there is no one *whose* illusion the conscious self could be, no one *who* is confusing herself with anything' (Metzinger 2003, p. 634).

Tye's and Metzinger's mistake lie in confounding the phenomenal and the ontological aspects of self and using them in an interchangeable manner. For them, it is not a viable position to accept the ontological aspect of the self.

7.2.1 Is Qualia Impersonal?

Representationalists endorse the impersonal characteristic of qualia. This is not true in our real, lived life. Sensations come to us not in a blank, receptor mode. The unique features of our personalities are the filters through which they arrive, change, and sustain. The implications of the feel factor is different for each person. Feel is not an isolated, clear, cognitive event. It is much more subjective in the sense it involves mood changes, invokes memories, and even brings in value-abidance in life. The phenomenal aspects of an experience can transform a person for good or bad. Hence, the result or the extent of the feel can continue for several days, indefinitely, or stay just for that moment.

Following Nagel (1974) and others before him, we curiously ask 'what it is like' to have a specific experience that belongs to another being. The mystery of 'what it is like' sustains since we tend to address it in a cognitive context. With such an address the wholesome character of experience is reduced or ignored. The query 'what it is like to be someone' is about subjectivity and being as a whole, in its uniqueness.

The query on subjectivity as a whole is distinct from two other queries:

(a) What it is like to eat sushi?
(b) What it is like to experience the flavour of sushi enjoyed by A?

(a) is about the experience of a distinct sensation and (b) is about the distinct feelings that A enjoys from the flavour. (a) Is object-centred. (b) Is person-centred.

Is (a) equivalent to (b)?

Unless we make this distinction, the larger question of 'what it is like to be oneself' cannot be approached. Nagel remarks: '… the analogical form of the English expression 'what it is *like*' is misleading. It does not mean 'what (in our experience) it *resembles*', but rather 'how it is for the subject himself' (Nagel 1974).

7.3 Feeling and its Uniqueness

Each discrete sensation comes with its designated feel. The feel of touch is different from the feel of watching sunset (and touch itself has myriad nuances depending on a large number of factors). The feel of anger is different from both these. What this means is that each sensation and mental state is discretely experienced. However, we cannot say that the feel is a property of the object of experience. We can only presume that the feel is a property of subjective experiences invoked by the object.

Yet another issue is about the universality of feel. When we endure a toothache, or drink coffee, or watch the redness of an evening sky, these experiences invoke a certain element of discomfort (in the case of toothache), or joy (in the case of watching sunset), or another unique feel. The feel factor is dependent on the object and the personality of its beholder. The nature of the feel invoked by the objects has universal accompanying features such as ownership and an assuring sense of being related to the experienced world. But the consequences of feel need not be the same for all. For instance, I may become irritated upon my toothache and go through a bad mood the whole day. Or I may quietly watch the discomfort without being overwhelmed by it.

Feel cannot be considered in isolation as a one-time experience. Feel is fully comprehended only if the one-time experience is extended to include the consequences such a feel produces in terms of attitudinal responses. The feel factor is guided by the reflective consciousness the self possesses. At any case, what is arguably confirmed is that there is a subjective feel to human experience. The feel has unique nuances exclusive to the person, as well as universal features that influence the experience, the experiencer, and the cohabitants in an interpersonal world.

A few philosophers have argued that consciousness is not a composite and unitary entity but discrete and formed of different states. One such view holds thus:

> When philosophers and psychologists think about consciousness, they generally focus on one or more of three features: phenomenality, intentionality, and introspectibility. I argue that, rather than being three features of a single, noncompositestate, these three features characterize different states of human beings. ... And because each feature characterizes an important way in which things like human beings differ from things like rocks, no one state has any more priority in being considered as what consciousness really is than the others (although the consciousness that most firmly grounds our personhood is probably introspectibility, where 'personhood' is that property that grounds moral agency....
>
> Each of intentionality, phenomenality, and introspection is a state we possess and rocks or roses do not. If consciousness is what distinguishes us from such things, then, if the proposed theory is correct, each of these states has the same priority for being called 'consciousness'. ...Moreover, that these are three independent, dissociable states (though they sometimes causally interact) means that we should expect to find beings who do not possess all three states, but possess only some subset of them. It is very likely that some nonhuman animals are just such creatures. So my philosophical theory begins to edge into a scientific one insofar as it has testable consequences. To the question, 'But what about the unity of consciousness?' I reply that there is no unity, only the appearance of it (Nelkin 1993, pp. 419, 432).

The discussion on feel demonstrates to us that in fact consciousness *is* marked by its unity, and its intentional, phenomenal and introspective capabilities come together. What offers serious challenges to the unidirectional and closed theories about feel and its relation to sensation is the poser, 'Can sensations be altered'? Can perceptions happen without a feel? Is there a possibility for brain to transfer and switch over sensory functions? Is feel a natural state or is it induced? If so, what is the nature of the subjective self that gives a coherent feel about sensations? By establishing the irreducible feel factor in all experiences, can we argue for an irreducible self?

Arguments for the non-reducibility of feel are often demonstrated with thought experiments. The 'Mary's knowledge' argument[2] (Jackson 1977), and 'what it is like to be a bat'[3] argument (Nagel 1974) make strong cases for the existence of qualia. Yet another thought experiment to favour the subjective irreducibility of qualia is the fictional instrument called the 'autocerebroscope' suggested by Feigl (1967). Though in a macabre manner, it helps make a strong argument for the independent existence of feel. The autocerebroscope is a hypothetical brain scanner with which you can look into your brain and see the neural firings for your experiences. The experiment implies the limitations of causal relations in explaining the connections between neural processes and the actual experience.

---

[2] The 'Mary's knowledge' argument is a thought experiment that refutes physicalism, and states that in spite of the availability of all the objective physical facts of colour vision, the scientist Mary did not know what it was to experience colour vision until she moved to the real world from the confinement of a black-and-white room.

[3] Nagel argues in this famous paper that subjective quality is central to consciousness.

Feinberg explains the thought experiment:

> There is a viewer attached to the probe with a magnification device that allows you to observe the neurons of your own brain. Suppose one day, as you are merrily viewing your brain, you come upon your thalamus, the source of your feeling of pain. Suddenly you sneeze, and the scope's eyepiece pokes you in the eye! You now experience intense pain while you are looking through the scope at the very neurons in the thalamus that created that pain. Now you ask yourself: Did you see anything through your autocerebroscope that was equal to the pain that you experienced? Was there anything that you observed that explained your pain? You surely saw the neurons responsible for your pain, and you could analyze the brain chemistry of these neurons, but does this allow you to reduce your pain to those neurons? It was your neurons themselves, not your image of the neurons through the viewer, that hurts! It occurs to you that there appears to be a gap between the neurons as they are observed by you and the neurons themselves as they are experienced by you within your brain. And you cannot find the source of this difference no matter how long and hard you observe your brain and think about the thalamus (Feinberg 2001, p. 145).

The unbridgeable epistemic gap between observing a brain in a feeling state and being a brain in the feeling state seems to only increase. How and why does brain activity generate feeling? The problem is not how specific patterns of brain activity are generated but how *feeling itself* is generated (Harnad 2005). The feel factor is inevitable, The neural description of a particular feel is incomplete without the actual experience. Further, it is not even possible to chart a clear pathway that begins with the physicality of neural structures and ends with the subjectivity of the experience. Perhaps this is the reason why Chalmers preferred to call qualia the 'hard problem' of consciousness.

7.3.1 Making Sense of Mixed up Senses

Are the 'how' and 'when' (correlates) of feelings neurally determined? Is the brain hard-wired for each sensation separately and without change? Does the brain differentiate senses always? Can there be cross-sensory experiences? Can the conscious agent intervene and adapt to such experiences? Does the feel factor always follow sensation and not vice versa? The case studies in synesthesia (Ramachandran 1998; Cytowic 2002) and experiments in auditory vision invoke these questions and challenge our classical idea about the feel defined by sensation.

In usual conditions, we experience our five senses discretely. But what if the causes and effects of sensations are mixed up? Synesthesia[4] involves a breakdown in communication between areas within the brain, leading to a release of limbic processes which are, in turn, experienced as synesthetic percepts (Cytowic 2002). It is a perceptual condition of mixed sensations. A stimulus in one sensory modality

---

[4] The word 'anesthesia' means 'no sensation'. 'Synesthesia' means 'joined sensation' (Greek, *syn* = together; *aisthesis* = perception). Synesthesia may also be induced by sensory deprivation, hallucinogens such as LSD and peyote, or direct electrical stimulation of subcortical limbic structures.

involuntarily elicits a sensation in a different sense, or senses. An internal intentional object is constructed during perception (Cytowic 2002, p. 350) without a corresponding external object of reference. Synesthetes also experience mixed sensations with the same modality. For instance, perception of a form may induce the perception of colour.

In his historic work, *Synesthesia: A union of the senses*, Cytowic (2002) details the extensive studies he undertook to find the basis of synesthesia. What is pertinent in synesthesia, according to Cytowic, is the prominence of intense emotion and strong beliefs. Synesthetic percepts, according to him, are neither a conventional perception nor an image. They possess a curious spatial extension and dynamism, and are involuntary, automatic, and consistent over time (Cytowic 2002, p. 33). Synesthesia is abnormal only in being statistically rare. He argues that synesthesia is possibly a normal brain process that is prematurely displayed to consciousness in a minority of individuals. Is the brain adaptive to our efforts to replenish it with sensory content on the wake of the fail of one sensory modality? The case of synesthesia suggests the possibility.

The mixing up of sight with sound (chromesthesia) is by far the most frequent synesthetic experience. Colour, movement and geometric shape are typical properties of the synesthete's sensations. For persons endowed with coloured hearing, for example, speech and music are not only heard but also a visual mélange of coloured shapes, movement and scintillation is experienced (Cytowic 2002, p. 16). The narration of the strange experiences that a synesthete could have baffles us and questions our taken-for-granted notions about normality, beliefs, discrete sensory experiences and body responses that we think we have naturally.

Studies also show that emotion and the limbic system have a greater role in synesthesia. Emotion, in fact, has a significant role in normal sensory function. Ramachandran's example of the sounds 'buba' and 'kiki' (Ramachandran 1998) that give an image of smoothness and ruggedness to the listener encourages us to consider if we have the natural ability to add emotional valence to sounds in everyday life.

Works by Peter Meijer describes how the blind are helped through auditory vision, which is seeing with sound (Sandhana 2003). The device is a tiny camera, a laptop and headphones. The camera is mounted on the head and the laptop takes the video input and converts it into auditory information, or 'soundscapes'. The scene in front is scanned in stereo. The object on the left is heard through the subject's left ear and the object on the right is heard through their right ear. Brightness is translated as volume. Bright things are louder. Pitch tells the subject what is up and what is down. The image refreshes once a second (Motluk 2005).

Efforts continue to locate the responsible neural region, and explore the potential, of auditory vision. An announcement from *Neuroreport* says that identifying objects with a visual-to-auditory sensory substitution device is associated with activation of occipital visual areas (Merabet et al. 2009). When one identifies an object's shape, a particular part of the brain called the lateral-occipital tactile-visual area (LOtv) is activated. At first this area was thought to be purely visual. Amedi Stern and others have shown that touch and hearing could also activate it (Stern et al. 2007). One can touch and 'see' a shape. One can hear and 'see' a shape.

Amedi suggests a significant finding that the brain is ultimately not interested in the *mode* of input as much as we assume generally. The brain is driven by the *presence* of an object. Whether the input is visual, tactile, or auditory is not reckoned.

The instances narrated above imply that feel is not strictly pre-designated with a sense organ. What we can assume is that there is a feel factor (due to the presence or absence of a sensation) that influences the brain to behave differently either by natural disposition (as in the case of synesthesia) or by non-invasive techniques such as auditory vision. These instances question our standard ways of understanding the working of brain. They also bring to light the place of the human self that constantly challenges the brain, and seeks adaptability to neural changes, through will power, urge to experience, the hope to live better, and emotional richness.

7.4 Emotions and the Self

Mainstream neuroscience and neuropsychiatry tend to favour a cybernetic view of human personality where sensation, awareness and experience are tools for humans to interact with the environment, and improve based on the feedback received from sensations. The standard view about the human brain emerges from the position that brain areas and functions can be chartered, and that the brain behaves in hierarchical order with the neocortex in lead. Sense organs perceive and produce sensations. The mind builds concepts. The brain puts them together through formal computational configurations, linguistic rules, and labelling. Much of the works in cognitive sciences take this as the standard view.

Is not this itself a poor concept—to divide brain and human capacities into sensations and concepts? Are we just machine like entities performing only rule-based cognitive tasks? Is not being a human much to do with the emotions and feelings we give and take, the worries and joys we experience, the hopes and expectations we cherish, the values and visions we build, the constant exploration we engage in to know our true selves?

Richard Cytowic writes:

> … it is linear and therefore something like a machine. The metaphoric likening of the brain, reason, and the mind to a machine is well known and extensively written about. The concept of hierarchy makes the cortex the brain's most important part. This part of the standard view says that the cortex is where consciousness, mind, reason, and reality are all located, and that everything below it is literally subservient. An important corollary says that language is the supreme cortical function; therefore, introspection, which is our self-conscious internal talking to ourselves, is a valid way to understand everything that goes on in our minds. Introspection has a long history in the philosophy of mind, but I will show its severe limitations and that we actually have several concurrent streams-of-consciousness running every moment (Cytowic 2002, p. 25).

In recent times, there is greater interest to bring such a position to scrutiny. This interest has been favoured by the narratives and case studies neuropsychiatrists share with the world. The documentation of medical cases, though, is a practice that existed since a very long time, books and works produced in the current and last decade particularly take the novel method of storytelling. And, we have a penchant to listen to stories, especially when they are about the strange and curious experiences of our fellow beings. Cashing on our innate interest in listening about ourselves, the works come in with interesting titles from Oliver Sacks, Jonathan Cole and others, which would qualify for literary imagination.

Many of these titles, even when they hold on to a hardcore neural and evolutionary description of the self, leave an open space to wonder if the self will ever become amenable to neural laws and explanations. The persistence to hold on to neural reductionism is best seen in the efforts to simplistically label certain cortical areas to be the locus of nuanced emotions and self-expressions. Temporal lobes get to be the deciding factor of all that which we express and have in terms of emotion and imagination; and of course dysfunctions to these as well.

Self in many of these discussions is only a placeholder for reference to put the discrete functions into a cohered whole. Terms such as ‘synaptic self’, ‘proto-self’, ‘narrative self’, ‘autobiographical self’, ‘enduring self’ etc. are used to explain the neural basis of self.

Ramachandran writes:

> … enduring self, is neither a separable subject of consciousness nor a homunculus, but it can be mapped anatomically to limbic and other associated structures which ‘drive’ frontal executive processes.… Even though the notion of a unitary, enduring self may turn out to be a form of adaptive self-deception or delusion … we must consider why the illusion arises (Ramachandran and Hirstein 1997, pp. 430, 454).

According to Metzinger:

> It is just a way of experiencing reality: currently, you *are* someone. What makes consciously experienced selfhood special, and different from all the other forms of experiential content, is the fact that—in nonpathological standard situations and in beings like ourselves—it is highly invariant. It is *always* there (Metzinger 2003, p. 626).

Damasio has certainty about the veracity of neural explanations but quibbles:

> … consciousness is the process whereby a mind is imbued with a reference we call self, and is said to know of its own existence and of the existence of objects around it (Damasio 1994, p. 192).

> A friend of mine who follows the developments of biology with keen interest and is an equally avid seeker of the spiritual in life often asks me if the spirit can be defined and located in neurobiological terms. ‘What is the spirit?’‘Where is it?’ How can I answer? I must confess I do not favor the attempt to neurologize religious experiences, especially when the attempts take the form of identifying a brain center for God or justifying God and religion by finding their correlates in brain scans. Yet, spiritual experiences, religious or otherwise, are mental processes. They are biological processes of the highest level of complexity. They occur in the brain of a given organism in certain circumstances and there is no reason why we should shy away from describing those processes in neurobiological terms provided we are aware of the limitations of the exercise (Damasio 2003, p. 284).

The working definitions of the self proposed by Ramachandran, Metzinger, Damasio and others inspire us to ask further questions. On what premises can we conclude that the self is a delusion caused by the neural circuitry, and not the rest of the concepts we build or the experiences we have? What is the benchmark for that distinct judgement? Are our 'normal' behaviours and life expressions interesting only to that extent that they are not pathological? If we pre-concede the limitations of a method in advance then how can we claim veracity and finality for its hypotheses? Responses to these questions are answered to a great extent by the studies on the brain in the context of the emotional and social self. And, the central idea that comes through is that *the self is challenged by the brain and the brain is challenged by the self.*

For Damasio, for instance, spiritual experiences are biological and mental processes of highest level of complexity. To describe them in neurobiological terms has its limitations. But the efforts have to continue. The self and the brain mutually reinforce at all times. We might say that to delimit the connections to wholly neurological, mental or spiritual domains will be to put the cart behind the horse. Perhaps, the tentative truths about each lie in their interactions with the other.

7.4.1 Emotions that Reason

In technical discussions we tend to discriminate reason and its abilities to be the arbitrator to judge the 'objectivity' of a thought expressed in words. Many a times we take thinking to be a rational process and accordingly rate how people think. But is all of thinking reason-based? Are our thoughts distinctly rational when we make decisions or make a judgement, or make a preference?

Not quite! Our thoughts are influenced by our whole personalities and not just discrete reason-based calculations and assessments. The overall nature of thinking is not directed by a well-organized system of reason and its attributes, but biased by the attributes of the person who thinks the thoughts. Fears, desires, expectations, frustrations, joys, intuitions, values and emotions frame even a very rationally expressed thought. The only reason that such a complexity driving a thought is not very visible in its expression is because reason is influenced by subliminal tendencies sometimes not apparent even for the thinker. A mathematician writes:

> Reasoning is the kind of thinking that can be coherently expressed in words, so useful for all kinds of communication and memorization. But thinking is more than reasoning: there is a vast complex of interpolation, extrapolation, interpretation, association, habits and illusions, to name but a few issues. The cooperation of all these intangible things, sometimes referred to as intuition, may finally produce ideas that can be expressed by words. Most ideas are not produced by reasoning alone (Bruijn 1996, p. 431).

Mainstream studies in cognitive sciences focus on reason-driven qualities of consciousness. When even a subject matter such as the feel is studied in an exclusively rational fashion, Damasio's and Ledoux's (2002) approach to integrate emotion into the study of the self is noteworthy, though the method is mostly biological. Damasio considers consciousness and emotions as states of the body, more specifically, of the immune system. He uses Cartesian dualism as a point of departure. He argues, based on neuroscientific research, that reason and emotion are closely linked and at the same time distinguishes feelings from emotions

(Damasio 1999). There have also been studies arguing that even aesthetic emotion and aesthetic pleasure can be related to cognitive experience (Pouivet 2000).

Emotion is physical. Feeling is mental. For Damasio, emotions are neural processes that respond to a stimulus. Emotion is the reaction for a stimulus to choose flight-or-fight options. It is also responsible for the homeostatic regulation. Here, too, a similar question arises as in the case of qualia. If all that is meant by qualia is that which automatically provides organisms with survival-oriented behaviours, then why is a subjective feel involved in emotion? Homeostasis and response to stimulus can happen without generating a subjective emotion. But on the contrary, the influence of emotions is complex, in the words of Damasio himself, who formulates a reductive biological theory of emotions and consciousness.

> In organisms equipped to sense emotions, that is, to have feelings, emotions also have an impact on the mind, as they occur, in the here and now. But in organisms equipped with consciousness, that is, capable of knowing they have feelings, another level of regulation is reached. Consciousness allows feelings to be known and thus promotes the impact of emotion internally, allows emotion to permeate the thought process through the agency of feeling. Eventually, consciousness allows any object to be known—the 'object' emotion and any other object—and, in so doing, enhances the organism's ability to respond adaptively, mindful of the needs of the organism in question. Emotion is devoted to an organism's survival, and so is consciousness (Damasio 1999, p. 35).

According to James (1884) and Damasio, feeling is a mental representation or mental map of the bodily state. Feeling is mental awareness whereas emotion is its visible effect. Emotion is physical and precedes feeling, which is mental. Emotion results in a physical behaviour and creates a neural map, which in turn leads to the feeling. A few scholars argue that there could also be what is called unconscious emotions, even though Freud did not attribute the unconscious nature to emotion but only to its cause.

> Emotions are not always felt. When emotion is felt, the feeling is a emotion: the emotion is a conscious perception of a patterned change in the body. But emotions can go unfelt: they can be unconscious perceptions of patterned changes in the body (Prinz 2005, p. 17).

Emotions can also involve imagined perceptions.

> A real life emotional experience involves perceptions, thoughts and feelings, typically directed towards the object of the emotion. Recognition that one is having an emotional experience is not necessary a part of every such experience. So, if an emotional experience where to have an imaginative counterpart, then we would expect it to involve *imagined* perceptions, thoughts and feelings typically directed towards the *imagined* object (Goldie 2005, p. 131).

Can affective and cognitive processes be distinctly conceptualized? Jaak Panksepp argues in the affirmative with the suggestion for different locales for their origin and processing, based on the studies of animals.

> Affects have a neo-cortical locus of control; they arise from broad-scale *state control* functions—large scale neural ensembles in action; they are analog, less computational, and generate *intentions-in action* that guide *action-to-perception* processes, with many neuropeptidergic codes. In contrast cognitions have a neocortical locus of control; they arise from more discrete informational *channel informations*. Thus cognitions are more

> digital, more computational, can generate *perception-to-action* processes that can lead to *intentions-to-act*, and are profoundly dependent on rapidly acting amino-acid transmitters (Panksepp 2005, pp. 173–174).

The cognition-emotion divide is presented in terms of somatic and felt differences by Damasio. Damasio echoes William James' idea that we first react with the body and then we feel. James talks about the transition from an 'object-simply-apprehended', through the sense organ, to an 'object-emotionally-felt'.

> A purely disembodied human emotion is a nonentity.... [E]motion dissociated from all bodily feeling is inconceivable.... [E]motion is nothing but the feeling of the reflex bodily effects of what we call its 'objects,' effects due to the connate adaptation of the nervous system to that object.... [E]motion both begins and ends with what we call its effects or manifestations. It has no mental *status* except as either the presented feeling, or the idea, of the manifestations.... An object falls on a sense-organ and is apperceived by the appropriate cortical center; or else the latter, excited in some other way, gives rise to an idea of the same object. Quick as a flash, the reflex currents pass down through their pre-ordained channels, alter the condition of muscle, skin and viscus; and these alterations, apperceived like the original object, in as many specific portions of the cortex, combine with it in consciousness and transform it from an object-simply-apprehended into an object-emotionally-felt (James 1884, pp. 193, 203).

Developing the view of James on the bodily origin of emotion, a key hypothesis Damasio offers is the 'somatic marker' (Damasio 1994), which highlights the importance of emotional learning in making effective decisions. There is an important role for feelings in reasoning. In a given situation feelings enable us to narrow down the number of possible choices for an action. It helps us with consequential thinking and cautions about high risk actions. The idea of somatic markers, according to Damasio, also has potential benefits in therapies for mental health.

> Knowing about emotion, feeling, and their workings does matter to how we live. At the personal level, this is quite certain. Within the next two decades, perhaps sooner, the neurobiology of emotion and feelings will allow biomedical science to develop effective treatments for pain and depression grounded on a sweeping understanding of how genes are expressed in particular brain regions and how these regions cooperate to make us emote and feel. Combined with psychological interventions, the novel therapies will revolutionize mental health (Damasio 2003, p. 184).

With the help of historical medical cases[5] and his own case studies, Damasio (1999) demonstrates that impairment to the pre-frontal cortical area (according to him, this is the seat of 'somatic markers') also impairs the ability to use reason or behave rationally. In short, to make rational decisions we need feelings as well. Emotion and feeling are equally important for the neural machinery, and are the

[5] Phineas Gage (1823–1860) is one of the earliest documented cases of severe brain injury which led to significant findings. An accident destroyed areas of his prefrontal lobe, and consequentially led to loss of his emotional and social capacities. His rational capabilities were intact to some extent. The damage interfered with Gage's capacity for planning and deciding a course of action. Damasio also narrates the case of Elliot who had a medical condition that affected the frontal lobe. He suffered from poor judgement and lack of insight, though he excelled in IQ tests. Patients like Gage and Elliot, though they perform well in cognitive and intelligence tests, show marked deficits in decision-making in everyday life.

foundation for biological regulations based on homeostatic controls. Neural processes and functions that are behind these mechanisms are distributed over several locations in the brain; their simultaneous working contributes to psychological phenomena. A reduction in emotion could contribute to irrational behaviour. Those with dysfunctions in decision-making seem to lack emotion, according to his studies.

Damasio's concept of emotion and the place he gives to the interconnections between feeling and reasoning are a welcome relief from the dominant theories that see the self as a computational or problem-solving process. Taking a different route from the notion that emotion is a remanence from the inheritance of the reptilian or the old mammalian brain, Damasio brings emotion into the forefront of sophisticated self-expressions and also proposes a theory of self. For Damasio, consciousness is a process whereby the mind gets the reference called self. Yet, for him to understand self is to understand its neural underpinnings and unravel the illusory sense of experience and its owner.

> … consciousness is the process whereby a mind is imbued with a reference we call self, and is said to know of its own existence and of the existence of objects around it. Elsewhere I have explained that in certain neurological conditions there is evidence that the mind process continues, but consciousness is impaired (Damasio 2003, p. 192).

> … overcoming the obstacle of self, which meant, from my standpoint, understanding its neural underpinnings, might help us understand the very different biological impact of three distinct although closely related phenomena: an emotion, the feeling of that emotion, and knowing that we have a feeling of that emotion (Damasio 1999, p. 10).

> … the neurobiology of consciousness faces two problems: the problem of how the movie-in-the-brain is generated, and the problem of how the brain also generates the sense that there is an owner and observer for that movie. The two problems are so intimately related that the latter is nested within the former (Damasio 1999, p. 12).

7.4.2 Illusory, but Emergent, Dimensional, and Layered Self

Given that he proposes the illusory nature of the self, one does not expect Damasio to go into the details of the different levels of the 'illusory' self. However, Damasio distinguishes between three kinds of self. There is an interconnected and temporarily coherent collection of neural patterns. These patterns represent the state of the organism, moment by moment, at multiple levels of the brain. This is the unconscious proto-self. The next level is the core-self, which is produced whenever an object of any kind modifies the proto-self. The core-self does not change much throughout our lifetime, and we are conscious of it.

Damasio relates his concept of core consciousness with the views expressed by earlier thinkers like Locke, Brentano, Kant, Freud, and William James. The third level is the autobiographical self, which is based on memory and anticipations of the future. It develops gradually throughout life. A core-self is needed in order to acquire an autobiographical self. But the core-self can exist without the autobiographical self. In certain cases of brain dysfunctions patients lose their autobiographical self, temporarily or permanently, while their core-self is intact.

> If core consciousness allows you to know for a transient moment that it is you seeing a bird in flight or that it is you having a sensation of pain, extended consciousness places these same experiences in a broader canvas and over a longer period of time. Extended consciousness still hinges on the same core 'you,' but that 'you' is now connected to the lived past and anticipated future that are part of your autobiographical record(Damasio 1999, p. 195).

The autobiographical self permits the existence of a richer form of consciousness—that Damasio calls extended consciousness—which is responsible for 'conscience' the highest level in this order. Though for Damasio the self is a biological re-construction and mind is the body, the layers of the self that he proposes seem to be borne of more imagination than biological reductionism. It is also clear that on the one hand Damasio presents a biologically defined self with emotion meant for biological survival; and on the other, his concept of self and consciousness bears the stamp of an artist or a person who imagines and believes in deeper and finer aspects of self. He writes:

> ... consciousness is the critical biological function that allows us to know sorrow or know joy, to know suffering or know pleasure, to sense embarrassment or pride, to grieve for lost love or lost life. Whether individually experienced or observed, pathos is a by-product of consciousness and so is desire. None of those personal states would ever be known to each of us without consciousness.
>
> Consciousness is, in effect, the key to a life examined,... knowing all about the hunger, the thirst, the sex, the tears, the laughter, the kicks, the punches, the flow of images we call thought, the feelings, the words, the stories, the beliefs, the music and the poetry, the happiness and the ecstasy. At its simplest and most basic level, consciousness lets us recognize an irresistible urge to stay alive and develop a concern for the self. At its most complex and elaborate level, consciousness helps us develop a concern for other selves and improve the art of life (Damasio 1999, pp. 7–8).

7.5 Sense, Sensations and Sensibilities

Within the area of self and consciousness studies the primary aspect of emotion that is discussed with relevance is the feel factor or the qualia of the experience. What makes an experience unique to the person defines its qualia and therefore it is mostly inaccessible to others. The closest relative to qualia is emotion because of its person-centric nature. Emotion, for neuroscience, is today one of the junctions where brain and personal experience meet. Yet, what is emotion is variously interpreted as brain states, bodily states, behaviours, feelings, cognitions, social roles, cultural practices, or any combination of these (Russell and Barrett 2009).

Apart from contributing to the qualia of experience emotions are those affective systems that are complex in terms of their actual experience, and its presentation within a theory of universal acceptance. While many have attempted definitions of emotion, the universal features for a mental state to be qualified as emotion are: cognitive antecedents, intentional objects, physiological arousal, physiological expressions, valence, and action tendencies (Elster 1998, p. 49). Emotions are *about something* and have intentional objects. They are recognized by observable expressions, and produce a valence, and action. Affective feelings tell us that something has intrinsic value (Gallagher and Panksepp 2008, p. 107). While keeping these universal features of emotion in mind, we also should remember that till date there has been less progress in generating a consensual definition for emotion.

> The struggle to define 'emotion' in scientific terms is as old as the field of psychology.... Izard's survey (2010) canvassed prominent emotion theoriests and researchers on their working definitions of emotion. The particular assumptions about emotion reported, as well as the conclusion that the term 'emotion' lacks a consensus definition, both have historical precedent.... [R]eviews have failed to identify the scientific criteria that distinguish one emotion from the next, or even emotions from cognitions....Izard's survey provides an important cautionary message to those who wish to treat 'emotion' as a scientific construct (Gendron 2010, pp. 371–372).

The study of emotions and emotional experiences has a history that takes us to the fascinating accounts of Charles Darwin (1872) in the West and Bharata (ca first century CE) in the East. While Bharata, through *Natyasastra*, his magnum opus of theatrics and aesthetics, discussed the pervasive nature of emotions, their empirical expressions and states of origin, Darwin focused mainly on some of the basic emotions such as fear, from the observations he made during his voyages.

The Western taxonomies of emotion are more similar to the *Natyasastra* taxonomy for negative than for positive emotions (Hejmadi et al. 2000, p. 183). What is noteworthy, but hardly referred to in an historical account of the study of emotions, is Bharata's underlying view that vision, movement, felt feelings, and expressed emotions are tied to the artist not just in an aesthetic sense but in both somatic and spiritual ways. The artist's self experiences an engagement coupled with detachment. Their agency brings in control of the somatic configurations, emotional expressions, while being in receptive awareness for sensory and mental information from themselves and the audience.

A similar understanding is reported from a recent study of ballet dancers, which considers agency to be tied up with control, receptivity and transformation (Legrand and Ravn 2009), and subjectivity to exist in movement. While our movement and gait are influenced and changed by emotional and other mental content at the prevailing time (Crane et al. 2006); amplitude, speed and fluidity of movement and gesture are indicators of underlying emotional process (Castellano et al. 2007); Studies have also established that emotions can be recognized through multiple modalities such as face, body gesture and speech (Castellano et al. 2008). A cluster of studies presented at the 2012 Alzheimer's Association's International Conference in Vancouver have linked physical changes such as changes in gait, to early signs before cognitive impairments manifest (Paddock 2012).

Emotion influences our body and subjectivity. The reverse also might be true to a certain extent that the expressions on our face, and the style of motion we adopt also reverse influence the emotions that could prevail. The exciting question from the mutual influence between emotion and body is whether emotion has a primary or intermediary role in actualizing the finer planes of self (Menon 2011). The ongoing discussion on whether we can agree upon a set of emotions as basic, and whether the rest of the emotions can be worked out from them is largely guided by the constituents of emotion itself than its impact upon the self.

It is a matter agreed upon by all of us that somehow our emotions have influences on our body and bodily organs. Our body and face represent the emotions felt, through different facial expressions, variations in temperature, and skin texture. A major debate in emotion studies is about the face and facial expressions. Darwin (1872) brought in the relevance of facial and bodily expressions into the light of scientific discussion in his 'The Expression of Emotions in Man and Animals'. Darwin asked why a particular expression was associated with a particular emotion, and the ensuing work formed part of his demonstration of the continuity of the species. The first major critique on 'emotional expression' and the antecedent place of emotion was given by Israel Waynbaum in 1907[6] who argued that the subjective experience of emotions follows the expression (muscular movement) of it. The crux of Waynbaum's theory is that behaviour, i.e. facial movements, precedes the experience of emotions that involve vascular changes. He postulated that stimuli trigger muscular movements that result in cerebral blood flow associated with facial emotional expressions.

Do the bodily expressions of emotion cause the subsequent experience of feeling an emotion, or does emotion cause movements and expressions of the body? This is a topic that has engaged psychologists, philosophers and physicians over the last century. A major attempt to trace the neural and anatomical correlates of emotions, primarily those that are described as 'self-conscious' emotions, such as embarrassment, pride and guilt (Dahlberg 2011), might also help explain the function of emotions in large to contribute to and shape social relations. The significant neural areas and anatomical systems that are watched upon to trace the route of emotions from chemical to psychological space of the self are the limbic system, thalamus, insula and pregenual anterior cingulate cortex. The downside of such approaches is the assumption that emotions are evolutionarily driven and hence biologically primitive. It is also to be critically examined if each emotion is biologically basic and is a separate, inherited, complex reflex that is hard-wired at birth (Barrett 2006a, p. 30).

A comparative and collative study of basic emotions and emotion systems (Ortony and Turner 1990) argues for affective valence, to feel positive or negative, to be the hallmark of an emotion. Emotion cannot be generating neutral valence (though according to Aristotle 'indifference' is also an emotion). Following this argument one could ask if complex psychological systems like desire can be moved out of the category of emotions. Geoffrey Madell (1997, p. 155) argues to the contrary: that some emotions are varieties of desire such as longing or yearning for something; and some emotions are varieties of pleasure such as joy and elation.

It might also be not fruitful to categorize all human experiences under the rubric of emotions. Emotions are not a collection of various psychological functions. Emotions are typically experienced as unified states of mind, rather than sets

[6] See: Zajonc, R. B. (1985, April 5) Emotion and facial efference: a theory reclaimed. *Science*, 228(4695): 15–21.

of components such as belief, desire, physiological perturbation, and some behaviour (Roberts 1988, p. 184). The pervasive attempt to distinguish emotion and feeling, or to address emotion as a composite of components, has also faced criticism. Another author on emotions, Robert Solomon, writes:

> … insofar as a feeling is valuable in analysing emotion, feeling and emotion are neither distinguishable nor independently specifiable.… [T]he sense of 'feeling' usually employed in the analysis of emotions is far too conceptually primitive to do justice to the richness and wisdom of our emotional lives (Solomon 1986, p. 654).

Another prominent approach towards emotions is to list a basic or fundamental set from which other emotions can be worked out. To trace a list of basic emotions, their neural correlates, and chart a singular biochemical route for the traverse of these highly phenomenal psychological phenomena might not aid in understanding their complex nature and existence. One of the reasons that emotion cannot be taken as an exclusive scientific category is that there does not seem to be a single feature that is always present in all emotional phenomena (Ledoux 1998). Arguing against enumerating a few as basic emotions, and building the rest from a finite number of basic constitutive elements, a strong position is that emotions, like languages, cannot have basic building blocks (Ortony and Turner 1990) and it favours a dimensional approach (Barrett and Wager 2006). These positions are in opposition with the naturalist explanation and the placement of emotions.

> The natural-kind view not only has shaped the kinds of scientific questions asked about emotion, but has also dictated how the evidentiary record should be interpreted. For example, if coordinated responses are the rule, then every instance of anger is supposed to produce a recognizable pattern of facial movements, vocal changes, peripheral nervous system activations, and voluntary behaviors. Instances in which responses do not coordinate are anomalies that require additional explanation (Barrett 2006a, b, p. 32).
>
> … [I]t is always appropriate to ask of those who propose basic emotions, 'What exactly do you mean? In what sense are you using the word 'basic'? What would count as empirical evidence for or against your claim, and why?' and 'What would you do with them if you had them?' We have suggested that current uses of the notion do not permit coherent answers to be given to such questions. More likely, the nearest one can come to some notion of ultimate basic emotions is that there are some basic classes of appraisals, such as the perception of an escapable or unescapable (sic) threat, that are associated with response patterns, such as fleeing or immobility, and that in some organisms, such responses, or better, the urge to produce them, occur in physiological, cognitive, phenomenal, and behavioral comples. It would be a cluster of such components that constitutes an emotion, rather than a single constituent of them, so that by the time these ingredients have combined to produce a full-fledged emotion, the notion of a basic emotion no longer applies. In this view, the complexity and the apparent limitlessness of different emotional feelings can be explained without recourse to a notion of basic emotions (Ortony and Turner 1990, p. 329).
>
> What are the basic building blocks of emotional life that a science of emotion should focus on? This question is almost as old as psychology itself, and it remains unanswered. The 'basic emotion' approach argues that certain categories of emotion, described by such English words as anger, sadness, fear, happiness, and disgust, are biologically basic—inherited, reflex-like modules that cause a distinct and recognizable behavioral and physiological pattern.… The ''dimensional' approach argues that anger, sadness, fear, and so on are categories that characterize more highly elaborated responses constructed from more fundamental, biological properties such as valence (pleasure/displeasure) and arousal (high activation/low activation…), positive and negative activation …, or approach and

> withdrawal…. The pressing question is which typology is given by nature and consists of 'natural kinds,' such that it is possible to make inductive discoveries about them? (Barrett and Wager 2006, p. 79).

Emotions are innumerable even when they are classified under social, counterfactual and positive or negative. An interesting classification made by a theorist considers 'cause' and 'belief' to be the deciding factor for the class to which an emotions belongs. He writes:

> Among the states that unambiguously qualify as emotions we may first list various social emotions: anger, hatred, guilt, shame, pride, pridefulness, admiration, and liking. Second there are various counterfactual emotions generated by thoughts about what might have happened but didn't: regret, rejoicing, disappointment, elation. Third, there are emotions generated by the thought of what may happen: fear and hope. Fourth, there are emotions generated by good or bad things that have happened: joy and grief. Fifth, there are emotions triggered by the thought of the possessions of others: envy, malice, indignation, and jealousy. Finally there are cases that do not fall neatly into any special category, such as contempt, dis-gust, and romantic love or 'limerence'. Borderline or controversial cases include surprise, boredom, interest, sexual desire, enjoyment, worry, and frustration. All of these emotions also allow for innumerable variations and nuances, depending on the exact nature of the beliefs that trigger them (Elster 1998, p. 48).

Elster further argues that most of the emotions are universal since their physiological and behavioural expressions are found in all societies, though some societies may lack a cognitive label for a given emotion. Referring to earlier works, he states instances such as: the notion of guilt did not exist in classical Greece; romantic love did not exist in Western Europe until the eleventh century (Elster 1998, p. 49). Hence, 'conceptualization of a state as an emotion is a necessary condition for that emotion to trigger meta-emotions as when we feel shame of envy or guilt about our anger' (p. 49).

7.6 The Inevitable Feel Factor

Is emotion an overall representation of our experience, or is it only one way of expressing an experience which is otherwise much more than mental? It is important to also consider the possibility of emotion being only a partial symbol of human experience. After all, our actions and experiences are driven by values, beliefs, commitments, and world views. The ancient but poignant Yogic theory does not even consider the class of emotions to categorize all of human experiences, but uses a much more universal structure of 'pain and pleasure' division. All experiences, according to Patanjali, can be classified under the resultant pain or pleasure. And in a later part of his text, he says, in fact even pleasurable experiences can be reduced to pain.

Emotions are pervasive phenomena interconnected with physiological mechanisms and phenomenal meanings in our daily lives. Emotions give us the feel factor through anatomical features (such as gut feelings) and psychological aspects. As unique individuals, we own and express different degrees of emotion, and thus some of us are described as 'warm' and some others as 'cold' in personality. Often, the degree of experience and expression of emotions is decided by the repertoire of our capabilities, dispositions such as our beliefs, desires, attention, and sensitivity to nuanced meanings, conceptualization and visualization.

A number of philosophical traditions both in the East and the West have nearly condemned emotions as obstructive agents in progress towards realizing the finer aspects of the self. At times, emotions are equated with outburst and uncontrolled behaviour that obstruct objective perception of situation. But often, without feeling emotions and expressing them, we cannot communicate with ourselves let alone others. The delicate nature of emotions aside, without feelings we cannot accurately assess the inner worlds of others and ourselves, cannot bring in creative and imaginative outpourings, and add enrichment to our personalities. The feel factor of emotion is the unavoidable face of consciousness whichever way it is conceived theoretically, as basic, or otherwise.

References

Arbib, M. A. (1989). *The metaphorical brain 2: Neural networks and beyond.* New York: Wiley-Interscience.

Arbib, M. A. (2002). In M. Richardson, R. J. Russell, P. Clayton, & K. Wegter-McNelly (Eds.), *The horrors of humanity and the computation of the self.* London: Routledge.

Armel, K. C., & Ramachandran, V. S. (2003). Projecting sensations to external objects: Evidence from skin conductance response. *Proceedings of the Royal Society of London: Biological, 270*, 1499–1506.

Aydin, K., Ucar, A., Oguz, K., Okur, O., Agayev, A., Unal, Z., et al. (2007). Increased gray matter density in the parietal cortex of mathematicians: A voxel-based morphometry study. *American Journal of Neurobiology, 28*, 1859–1864.

Barkovich, A. J., Millen, K. J., & Dobyns, W. B. (2009). A developmental and genetic classification for midbrain-hindbrain malformations. *Brain, 132*(12), 3199–3230.

Barrett, L. F. (2004). Feelings or words? Understanding the content in self-report ratings of experienced emotion. *Journal of Personality and Social Psychology, 87*, 266–281.

Barrett, L. F. (2006a). Are emotions natural kinds? *Perspectives on Psychological Science, 1*(1), 28–58.

Barrett, L. F. (2006b). Solving the emotion paradox: Categorization and the experience of emotion. *Personality and Social Psychology Review, 10*(1), 20–46.

Barrett, L. F., & Wager, T. D. (2006). The structure of emotion: Evidence from neuroimaging studies. *Current directions in Psychological Science, 15*(3), 79–83.

Barrett, L., Henzi, P., & Rendall, D. (2007). Social brains, simple minds: Does social complexity really require cognitive complexity? *Philosophical Transactions of the Royal Society: Biological Sciences: Social Intelligence: From Brain to Culture, 362*, 561–575.

Bayne, T. A. (2003). What is the unity of consciousness? In E. A. Cleeremans (Ed.), *The unity of consciousness: Binding, integration, dissociation* (pp. 23–27). Oxford: Oxford University Press.

Beauregard, V., & Paquette, M. (2006). Neural correlates of a mystical experience in Carmelite nuns. *Neuroscience Letters, 405*(3), 186–190.

Bermúdez, J. L. (2000). *The paradox of self-consciousness: Representation and mind.* Cambridge: MIT Press.

Bitbol, M., & Petitmengin, C. (2011). On pure reflection: A reply to Dan Zahavi. *Journal of Consciousness Studies, 18*(2), 24–37.

Blackmore, S. (1999). *The meme machine*. Oxford: Oxford University Press.

Blackmore, S. (2012). She won't be me. *Journal of Consciousness Studies, 19*(1–2), 16–19.

Blakeslee, S., & Blakeslee, M. (2008). *The body has a mind of its own: How body maps in your brain help you do (almost) everything better*. New York: Random House.

Bosco, F. M. (1998). Sharedness as an innate basis for communication in the infant. *Proceedings of the 20th Annual Conference of the Cognitive Science Society*. Mahwah: Erlbaum.

Botvinick, M., & Cohen, J. (1998). Rubber hand 'feels' touch that eyes see. *Nature, 391*, 756.

Brockman, J. (1997). *Organs of computation: A talk with Steven Pinker.* Retrieved 28 June 2012, from edge third culture: http://www.edge.org/3rd_culture/pinker/pinker_p1.html.

Bruijn, N. G. (1996). Can people think? *Journal of Consciousness Studies, 3*(5–6), 425–447.

Bruun, H., & Langlais, R. (2003). On the embodied nature of action. *Acta Sociologica, 46*(1), 31–49.

Castellano, G., Villalba, S., & Camurri, A. (2007). Recognising human emotions from body movement and gesture dynamics. In R. P. A. Paiva (Ed.), *Affective Computing and Intelligent Interaction, Second International Conference, ACII* 2007, *Lisbon* (Vol. 4738, pp. 71–82). Berlin: Springer.

Castellano, G., Kessous, L., & Caridakis, G. (2008). Emotion recognition through multiple modalities: Face, body gesture, speech. In *Lecture Notes in Computer Science: Affect and Emotion in Human-Computer Interaction* (Vol. 4868, pp. 92–103).

Chalmers, D. (1995). The puzzle of conscious experience. *Scientific American, 273*, 62–68.

Chalmers, D. (1999). *The scientific American book of the brain*. New York: The Lyons Press.

Chen, H., Cohen, P., Johnson, J., Kasen, S., Sneed, J., & Crawford, T. (2004). Adolescent personality disorders and conflict with romantic partners during the transition to adulthood. *Journal of Personality Disorders, 18*, 507–525.

Churchland, P. S., & Sejnowski, T. (1997). *The computational brain*. Cambridge: MIT Press.

Cole, J. (2004). *Still lives: Narratives of spinal cord injury*. Cambridge: MIT Press.

Cole, J. (2009). Impaired embodiment and intersubjectivity. *Phenomenology and the Cognitive Sciences, 8*(3), 343–360.

Costantini, M., & Haggard, P. (2007). The rubber hand illusion: Sensitivity and reference frame for body ownership. *Consciousness and Cognition, 16*, 229–240.

Cotterill, R. M. (2001). Evolution, cognition and consciousness. *Journal of Consciousness Studies, 8*(2), 3–17.

Coulter, J. (1979). The brain as agent. *Human Studies, 2*(4), 335–348.

Crane, E., Gross, M., & Fredrickson, B. (2006). Expression of emotion in body and face. *Proceedings of the 6th International Conference on Intelligent Virtual Agents* (p. 452).

Crick, F. (1995). *The astonishing hypothesis: The scientific search for the soul*. New York: Simon & Schuster.

Crick, F. H., & Koch, C. (1990). Toward a neurobiological theory of consciousness. *Seminars in the Neuroscience, 2*, 263–275.

Cytowic, R. (2002). *Synesthesia: A union of the senses*. Cambridge: Bradford.

Dahlberg, C. P. (2011). How embarrassing: Researchers pinpoint self-consciousness in the brain. *Scientific American*.

Damasio, A. (1994). *Descartes' error: Emotion, reason and the human brain*. New York: G. P. Putnam's Sons.

Damasio, A. R. (1998). Investigating the biology of consciousness. *Philosophical Transactions: Biological Sciences—The Conscious Brain: Abnormal and Normal, 353*(1377), 1879–1882.

Damasio, A. (1999). *Feeling of what happens: Body and emotion in the making of consciousness*. London: Heinemann.

Damasio, A. (2003). *Looking for Spinoza: Joy, sorrow and the feeling brain*. London: William Heinemann.

Daprati, E., Sirigu, A., & Nico, D. (2010). Body and movement: Consciousness in the parietal lobes. *Neuropsychologia, 48*, 756–762.

d'Aquili, E., & Newberg, A. (1993). Liminality, trance and unitary states in ritual and meditation. *Studia Liturgica, 23*, 2–34.
Darwin, C. (1872). *The expression of emotions in man and animals* (1st ed.). London: John Murray.
Davidson, R., & McEwen, B. (2012). Social influences on neuroplasticity: Stress and interventions to promote well-being. *Nature Neuroscience, 15*, 689–695.
Dawkins, R. (1976). *The selfish gene*. Oxford: Oxford University Press.
Deci, E. L., & Ryan, R. M. (2008). Hedonia, eudaimonia, and well-being: An introduction. *Journal of Happiness Studies, 9*, 1–11.
Dennett, D. (1991). *Consciousness explained*. London: Allen Lane.
Dennett, D. (1996). Facing backwards on the problem of consciousness. *Journal of Consciousness Studies, 3*(1), 4–6.
Diener, E. (1984). Subjective well-being. *Psychological Bulletin, 95*, 542–575.
Dimaggio, G., Lysaker, P., Carcione, A., Nicolo, G., & Semerari, A. (2008). Know yourself and you shall know the other... to a certain extent: Multiple paths of influence of self-reflection on mindreading. *Consciousness and Cognition, 17*, 778–789.
Dretske, F. (1995). *Naturalizing the mind*. Cambridge: MIT Press.
Edelman, G. M. (1998). Building a picture of the brain. *Daedalus: The Brain, 127*(2), 37–70.
Ellis, R. D. (2005). The roles of imagery and meta-emotion in deliberate choice and moral psychology. In G. Colombetti & E. Thompson (Eds.), *Journal of Consciousness Studies, 12*(8–10), 140–157.
Elster, J. (1998). Emotions and economic theory. *Journal of Economic Literature, 36*(1), 47–74.
Eriksson, P. S., Perfilieva, E., Björk-Eriksson, T., Alborn, A.-M., Nordborg, C., Peterson, D. A., et al. (1998). Neurogenesis in the adult human hippocampus. *Nature Medicine, 4*, 1313–1317.
Feigl, H. (1967). *The "mental" and the "physical"*. Minneapolis: University of Minnesota Press.
Feinberg, T. E. (2001). *Altered egos: How the brain creates the self*. Oxford: Oxford University Press.
Fields, J., Copp, M., & Kleinman, S. (2007). Symbolic interactionism, inequality and emotions. In J. E. Stets & J. H. Turner (Eds.), *Handbook of the sociology of emotions* (pp. 155–178). Berlin: Springer Science.
Foucault, M. (1988). *Technologies of the self*. In L. H. Martin, H. Gutman, & P. H. Hutton (Eds.), University of Massachusetts Press.
Franks, D. D. (2007). The neuroscience of emotions. In J. E. Stets & J. H. Turner (Eds.), *Handbook of the sociology of emotions* (pp. 38–62). Berlin: Springer Science.
Frederickson, B. (2001). The role of positive emotions in positive psychology: The broaden-and-build theory of positive emotions. *American Psychologist, 56*(3), 218–226.
Fuchs, T. (2011). The brain: A mediating organ. *Journal of Consciousness Studies, 18*(7–8), 196–221.
Gait Changes May Signal Cognitive Decline, Presage Alzheimer's. (2012). Retrieved from Medical News Today: http://www.medicalnewstoday.com/articles/247862.php.
Gallagher, S. (2000). Philosophical conceptions of the self: Implications for cognitive science. *Trends in the Cognitive Sciences, 4*(1), 14–21.
Gallagher, S. (2005). *How the body shapes the mind*. Oxford: Oxford University Press.
Gallagher, S. (2006). Where's the action? Epiphenomenalism and the problem of free will. In W. Banks, S. Pockett, & S. Gallagher (Eds.), *Does consciousness cause behaviour: An investigation of the nature of volition* (pp. 109–124). Cambridge: MIT Press.
Gallagher, S. (Ed.). (2011). *The Oxford handbook of the self*. Oxford: Oxford University Press.
Gallagher, S., & Cole, J. (1998). In D. Welton (Ed.), *Body and flesh: A philosophical reader*. Oxford: Blackwell.
Gallagher, S., & Marcel, A. (1999). The self in contextualized action. *Journal of Consciousness Studies, 6*(4), 4–30.
Gallagher, S., & Panksepp, J. (2008). How to undress the affective mind: An interview with Jaak Panksepp. *Journal of Consciousness Studies, 15*(2), 89–119.

Gallup, G. G. (1977). Self recognition in primates: A comparative approach to the bidirectional properties of consciousness. *American Psychologist, 32*(5), 329–338.

Gazzaniga, M. (2006). *The ethical brain: The science of our moral dilemmas*. New York: HarperCollins.

Gendron, M. (2010). Defining emotion: A brief history. *Emotion Review, 2*(4), 371–372.

Georgieff, N., & Jeannerod, M. (1998). Beyond consciousness of external reality: A "who" system for consciousness of action and self-consciousness. *Consciousness and Cognition, 7*, 465–477.

Goldie, P. (2005). Imagination and the distorting power of emotion. In G. Colombetti (Ed.) *Journal of Consciousness Studies, 12*(8–10), 127–139.

Greenberg, L. (2002). *Emotion-focused therapy: Coaching clients to work through feelings*. Washington: American Psychologist Association.

Hanson, R. (2011). *Institute of noetic sciences*. Retrieved 10 May 2012 from http://www.noetic.org/noetic/issue-nine-april/self-directed-neuroplasticity/.

Harman, W. (1994). The scientific exploration of consciousness: Towards an adequate epistemology. *Journal of Consciousness Studies, 1*(1), 140.

Harnad, S. (2005, January 13). *What is consciousness?* Retrieved from The New York Review of Books: http://www.nybooks.com/articles/archives/2005/jun/23/what-is-consciousness/.

Head, H. (1920). *Studies in neurology* (Vol. 2). London: Oxford University Press.

Heilman, K. M., Barrett, A. M., & Adair, J. C. (1998). Possible mechanisms of anosognosia: A defect in self-awareness. *Philosophical Transactions: Biological Sciences, 353*(1377), 1903–1909.

Hejmadi, A., Davidson, R., & Rozin, P. (2000). Exploring hindu Indian emotion expressions: Evidence for accurate recognition by Americans and Indians. *Psychological Science, 2*(3), 183–187.

Helmuth, L. (2002). Redrawing the brain's map of the body. *Science, New Series, 296*(5573), 1587–1588.

How Embarrassing: Researchers Pinpoint Self-Consciousness in the Brain. (2011). Retrieved from Scientific American Mind: http://www.scientificamerican.com/article.cfm?id=how-embarrassing&WT.mc_id=SA_DD_20111013.

Hume, D. (1947). In N. K. Smith (Ed.), *Dialogues concerning natural religion*. Edinburgh: Nelson.

Humphrey, N. (2006). *Seeing red: A study in consciousness*. Cambridge: The Belknap Press of Harvard University Press.

Iacoboni, M., Molnar-Szakacs, I., Gallese, V., Buccino, G., Mazziotta, J., & Rizzolatti, G. (2005). Grasping the intentions of others with one's own mirror neuron system. *PLoS Biology, 3*(3), 0529–0535.

Iyengar, S. S. (2000a). When choice is demotivating: Can one desire too much of a good thing? *Journal of Personality and Social Psychology, 79*(6), 995–1006.

Iyengar, S. S. (2000b). When choice is demotivating: Can one desire too much of a good thing? *Journal of Personality and Social Psychology, 79*(6), 1004.

Jackendoff, R. (1987). *Consciousness and the computational mind*. Cambridge: MIT Press.

Jackson, F. (1977). *Perception*. Cambridge: Cambridge University Press.

James, W. (1884). What is an emotion? *First published in Mind, 9*, 188–205.

James, W. (1890). *The principles of psychology*. Retrieved 7 Apr 2012, from Classics in the History of Psychology: http://psychclassics.asu.edu/James/Principles/prin10.htm.

James, W. (1985). In M. E. Marty (Ed.), *The varieties of religious experience: Edited with an introduction*. New York: Penguin Classics.

Joseph, R. (1990). *Neuropsychology, neuropsychiatry and behavioural neurology*. New York: Plenum Press.

Kandel, E. R., & Squire, L. R. (2000). Neuroscience: Breaking down scientific barriers to the study of brain and mind. *Science, 290*(5494), 1113–1120.

Kaufman, G. F., & Libby, L. K. (2012). Changing beliefs and behavior through experience-taking. *Journal of Personality and Social Psychology, 103*, 1.

Kelly, E. F., Kelly, E. W., Crabtree, A., Gauld, A., Grosso, M., & Greyson, B. (2007). *Irreducible mind: Toward a psychology for the 21st century*. Plymouth: Rowman and Littlefield Publishers Inc.
Kircher, T. T., & Leube, D. T. (2003). Self-consciousness, self-agency and Schizophrenia. *Consciousness and Cognition, 12*(4), 656–669.
Koch, C., & Greenfield, S. (2007). How does consciousness happen? *Scientific American, 297*, 50–57.
Kozart, M. (1998). Religious experience was not correctly defined. *Journal of Neuropsychiatry and Clinical Neurosciences, 10*, 475.
Kring, A. M. (2010). The future of emotion research in the study of psychopathology. *Emotion Review, 2*(3), 225–228.
Kupperman, J. J. (1991). *Character*. Oxford: Oxford University Press.
Kupperman, J. J. (1999). *Learning from Asian philosophy*. Oxford: Oxford University Press.
Langlitz, N. (2010). The persistence of the subjective in neuropsychopharmacology: Observations of contemporary hallucinogen research. *History of the Human Sciences, 23*(1), 37–57.
LeDoux, J. (1998). *The emotional brain: The mysterious underpinnings of emotional life*. New York: Simon & Schuster.
LeDoux, J. (2002). *Synaptic self: How our brains become who we are*. New York: Penguin Books.
Legrand, D., & Ravn, S. (2009). Perceiving subjectivity in bodily movement: The case of dancers. *Phenomenology and the Cognitive Sciences, 8*, 389–408.
Liviingston, P. (2002). Experience and structure: Philosophical history and the problem of consciousness. *Journal of Consciousness Studies, 9*(3), 15–33.
Lopez, C., Halje, P., & Blanke, O. (2008). Body ownership and embodiment: Vestibular and multisensory mechanisms. *Clinical Neurophysiology, 38*, 149–161.
Luria, A. (1968). *The mind of a mnemonist: A little book about a vast memory*. New York: Basic Books.
Lutz, A., Greischar, L. L., Rawlings, N. B., Ricard, M., & Davidson, R. J. (2004). Long-term meditators self-induce high-amplitude gamma synchrony during mental practice. *Proceedings of National Academy of Sciences, 101*(46), 16369–16373.
Lycan, W. G. (1995). *Consciousness*. MIT Press.
Lycan, W. G. (1996). *Consciousness and experience*. Cambridge: MIT Press.
Madell, G., & Ridley, A. (1997). Emotion and feeling. *Proceedings of the Aristotelian Society, Supplementary* (Vol. 71, pp. 147–176). Blackwell Publishing on behalf of the Aristotelian Society.
Maguire, E., Gadian, D., & Johnsrude, I. (2000). Navigation-related structural change in the hippocampi of taxi drivers. *Proceedings of the National Academy of the Sciences of the USA*, (pp. 4398–4403).
Majorek, M. B. (2012). Does the brain cause conscious experience? *Journal of Consciousness Studies, 19*(3–4), 121–144.
Manoussakis, J. P. (2007). *God after metaphysics*. Bloomington: Indian University Press.
McGinn, C. (1997). *The character of mind: An introduction to the philosophy of mind*. Oxford: Oxford University Press.
Menon, S. (2001). Towards a Sankarite approach to consciousness: A discussion in the context of recent interdisciplinary scientific perspectives. *Journal of Indian Council of Philosophical Research, 18*(1), 95–111.
Menon, S. (2002). Structure of mind and structured mind. *Indian Philosophical Quarterly, 2*(3), 335–344.
Menon, S. (2003). Binding experiences for a first person approach: Looking at Indian ways of thinking (darsana) and acting (natya) in the context of current discussions on 'consciousness'. In C. Chakraborti, M. K. Mandal, & R. B. Chatterjee (Eds.), *On mind and consciousness* (pp. 90–117). Shimla: Indian Institute of Advanced Study, Shimla and Department of Humanities and Social Sciences IIT Kharagpur.

Menon, S. (2009). The rain clouds of mind-modifications and the shower of transcendence: Yoga and Samadhi in Patanjali Yoga Sutra. In R. Rao (Ed.), *Yoga and parapsychology: Empirical research and theoretical essays* (pp. 169–199). Delhi: Motilal Banarsidass.

Menon, S. (2011). A first-person approach to aesthetic emotions in Natyasastra. In R. Narasimha & S. Menon (Eds.), *Nature and culture* (pp. 259–270). New Delhi: PHISPC and Centre for Studies in Civilisations.

Menon, S., & Bodhananda, S. (2003). *Dialogues: Philosopher meets seer*. New Delhi: Bluejay Books.

Merabet, L., Battelli, L., Obretenova, S., Maguire, S., Meijer, P., & Pascual-Leone, A. (2009). Functional recruitment of visual cortex for sound encoded object identification in the blind. *NeuroReport, 20*(2), 132–138.

Merleau-Ponty, M. (1964). *The primacy of perception*. Evanston: Northwestern University Press.

Metzinger, T. (2003). *Being no one: The self-model theory of subjectivity*. Cambridge: MIT Press.

Metzinger, T. (2009). *The ego tunnel: The science of the mind and the myth of the self.* New York: Basic Books.

Morison, R. S. (1983). Is there a biological person? *The Milbank Memorial Fund Quarterly: Health and Society: Special Issue: The Problem of Personhood: Biomedical, Social, Legal and Policy Views, 61*(1), 3–18.

Motluk, A. (2005). *Seeing with your ears*. New York: The New York Times.

Nagel, T. (1974). What is it like to be a bat? *Philosophical Review, 83*, 435–450.

Neisser, U. (1988). Five kinds of self-knowledge. *Philosophical Psychology, 1*(1), 35–59.

Nelkin, N. (1993). What is consciousness? *Philosophy of Science, 60*(3), 419–434.

Newberg, A., d'Aquili, E., & Rause, V. (2001). *Why god won't go away*. New York: Ballantine Books.

Nixon, G. M. (2012). You are not your brain: Against "teaching to the brain". In D. King, & K. Dyer (Eds.), *International Handbook of Academic Research and Teaching: Proceedings of Intellectbase International Consortium* (Vol. 22, pp. 298–306). San Antonio.

Nurius, P. S. (1993). Human memory: A basis for better understanding the elusive self-concept. *Social Service Review, 67*(2), 261–278.

Oberman, L. M., Hubbard, E. M., McCleery, J. P., Altschuler, E. L., Ramachandran, V. S., & Pineda, J. A. (2005). EEG evidence for mirror neuron dysfunction in autism spectrum disorders. *Cognitive Brain Research, 24*, 190–198.

Oltmanns, T. F., Gleason, M. E., Klonsky, E. D., & Turkheimer, E. (2005). Meta-perception for pathological personality traits: Do we know when others think that we are difficult? *Consciousness and Cognition, 14*, 739–751.

Ortony, A., & Turner, T. (1990). What's basic about basic emotions? *Psychological Review, 97*(3), 315–331.

Paddock, C. (2012). *Gait changes may signal cognitive decline, presage Alzheimer's*. Retrieved from Medical News Today: http://www.medicalnewstoday.com/articles/247862.php.

Panksepp, J. (2005). On the embodied neural nature of core emotional affects. In G. Colombetti, & E. Thompson (Eds.), *Journal of Consciousness Studies, 12*(8–10), 158–184.

Panksepp, J., Asma, S., Curran, G., Gabriel, R., & Greif, T. (2012). The philosophical implications of affective neuroscience. *Journal of Consciousness Studies, 19*(3–4), 6–48.

Parker, E. S., Cahill, L., & Mcgaugh, J. L. (2006). A case of unusual autobiographical remembering. *Neurocase, 12*, 35–49.

Patten, S. (1976). Hume's bundles, self-consciousness and Kant. *Hume Studies, 2*(2), 59–75.

Penfield, W. (1947). Ferrier lecture: Some observations on the cerebral cortex of man. *Proceedings of the Royal Society of London. Series B, Biological Sciences, 134*(876), 329–347.

Penfield, W. (1959). The interpretive cortex. *Science, New Series, 129*(3365), 1719–1725.

Penrose, R. (1994). *Shadows of the mind.* Oxford: Oxford University Press.

Petranker, J. (2003). Inhabiting conscious experience: Engaged objectivity in the first-person study of consciousness. *Journal of Consciousness Studies, 10*(12), 3–23.

Philippi, C. L., et al. (2012). Preserved self-awareness following extensive bilateral brain damage to the insula, anterior cingulate, and medial prefrontal cortices. *PLoS ONE, 7*(8), e38413.

Pile, S. (1993). Human agency and human geography revisited: A critique of 'new models' of the self. *Transactions of the Institute of British Geographers, 18*(1), 122–139.

Pinker, S. (1997). In J. Brockman (Ed.), *Organs of computation: A talk with Steven Pinker.* Retrieved 28 June 2012, from Edge Third Culture: http://www.edge.org/3rd_culture/pinker/pinker_p2.html.

Polanyi, M. (1966). *The tacit dimension*. London: The University of Chicago Press.

Porter, L. (2000). The bifurcated gift: Love and intimacy in drama psychotherapy. *The Arts in Psychotherapy, 7*(5), 309–320.

Pouivet, R. (2000). On the cognitive functioning of aesthetic emotions. *Leonardo, 33*(1), 49–53.

Premack, D. (1978). Does the chimpanzee have a theory of mind. *Behavioral and Brain Sciences, 1*, 512–526.

Prinz, J. (2005). Are emotions feelings? In G. Colombetti, & E. Thompson (Eds.), *Journal of Consciousness Studies, 12*(8–10), 9–25.

Ramachandran, V. A. (1998). *Phantoms in the brain*. New York: William Morrow.

Ramachandran, V. (2003). *The emerging mind*. London: The BBC in association with Profile Books Ltd.

Ramachandran, V., & Blakeslee, S. (1998). *Phantoms in the brain*. New York: William Morrow.

Ramachandran, V. S., & Hirstein, W. (1997). Three laws of Qualia: What neurology tells us about the biological functions of consciousness. *Journal of Consciousness Studies, 4*(5–6), 429–457.

Ramachandran, V. S., & Hirstein, W. (1998). The perception of phantom limbs: The D. *O. Hebb lecture. Brain, 121*(1), 1603–1630.

Reber, A. S. (1993). *Implicit learning and tacit knowledge: An essay on the cognitive unconscious*. New York: Oxford University Press.

Reid, T. (1994). In R. E. Beanblossom, & K. Lehrer (Eds.), *Inquiry and essays*. Indianapolis: Hackett.

Restak, R. M. (1982). The archaeology of the self. *The Wilson Quarterly, 6*(3), 98–104.

Restak, R. M. (1985). The human brain: Insights and puzzles. *Theory into Practise: Learning and the Brain, 24*(2), 91–94.

Rizzolatti, G., Fadiga, L., Gallese, V., & Fogassi, L. (1996). Premotor cortex and the recognition of motor actions. *Cognitive Brain Research, 3*, 131–141.

Robbins, A., Adler, S., Eigen, M., Roland, A., Strahl, L., & Wallace, E. (1979). Dialogue in creative and therapeutic growth. *Art Psychotherapy, 6*, 221–232.

Roberts, R. C. (1988). What an emotion is: A sketch. *The Philosophical Review, 97*(2), 183–209.

Rose, N. (2003). Neurochemical selves. *Society, 41*(1), 46–59.

Rosenfield, I. (1995). Memory and identity. *New Literary History: Narratives of Literature, the Arts, and Memory, 26*(1), 197–203.

Rosenthal, D. M. (2003). Unity of consciousness and the self. *Proceedings of the Aristotelian Society, New Series, 103*, 325–352.

Rudrauf, D., & Damasio, A. (2005). A conjecture regarding the biological mechanism of subjectivity and feeling. In G. Colombetti, & E. Thompson (Eds.), *Journal of Consciousness Studies, 12*(8–10), 236–262.

Russell, J. A., & Barrett, L. F. (2009). Editorial. *Emotion Review, 1*(1), 2.

Ryff, C. D. (1989). Happiness is everything, or is it? Explorations on the meaning of psychological well-being. *Journal of Personality and Social Psychology, 57*, 1069–1081.

Ryff, C., Singer, B., & Love, G. (2004). Positive health: Connecting well-being with biology. *Philoosphical Transactions*, 1383–1394.

Sacks, O. (1985). *the man who mistook his wife for a hat and other clinical tales*. New York: Summit Books.

Saks, E. R. (1999). *Interpreting interpretation: The limits of hermeneutic psychoanalysis*. New Haven: Yale University Press.

Sandhana, L. (2003, October 7). *Blind 'see with sound'*. Retrieved September 10, 2013, from BBC News: http://news.bbc.co.uk/2/hi/science/nature/3171226.stm.

Saver, J. L., & Rabin, J. (1997). The neural substrates of religious experiences. *Journal of Neuropsychiatry and Clinical Neurosciences, 9*(3), 498–510.

Schilder, P. (1950). *The image and appearance of the human body*. New York: International Universities Press.

Schwartz, J. M., & Begley, S. (2002). *The mind and the brain: Neuroplasticity and the power of the mental force*. New York: HarperCollins Publishers.

Scott Haig, M. (2007). The brain: The power of hope. *TIME*, 58–59.

Searle, J. (1995, November 2). The mystery of consciousness. *The New York Review of Books*, 63.

Searle, J. R. (2006). Minding the brain. *The New York Review of Books, LIII*(17), 51–55.

Searle, J. (2011, June 9). *The Mystery of Consciousness Continues*. Retrieved from The New York Review of Books: http://www.nybooks.com/articles/archives/2011/jun/09/mystery-consciousness-continues/.

Seligman, M. (2002). *Authentic happiness*. New York: Free Press.

Seth, A. K., Izhikevich, E., Reeke, G. N., & Edelman, G. M. (2006). Theories and measures of consciousness: An extended framework. *Proceedings of the National Academy of Sciences of the United States of America, 103*(28), 10799–10804.

Shanahan, D. (2008). A new view of language, emotion and the brain. *Integrative Psychological and Behavioural Science, 42*, 6–19.

Shear, J. (1996). The hard problem: Closing the empirical gap. *Journal of Consciousness Studies, 3*(1), 54–68.

Shear, J. (2007). Lecture on "Reflections on Embodiment" at the International Conference Titled "Body, Embodiment and Enworldment". Bangalore: National Institute of Advanced Studies.

Sherrington, C. S. (1906). *The integrative action of the nervous system*. New Haven: Yale University Press.

Shoemaker, S. (1994). The first-person perspective. *Proceedings and Addresses of the American Philosophical Association, 68*(2), 7–22.

Shoemaker, S. (2003). *Identity, cause, and mind: Philosophical essays*. Oxford: Oxford University Press.

Shoemaker, S., & Strawson, G. (1999). Self and body. *Proceedings of the Aristotelian Society, Supplementary Volumes, 73*, 287–332.

Simmel, M. L. (1958). The conditions of occurrence of phantom limbs. *Proceedings of the American Philosophical Society, 102*(5), 492–500.

Sloan, D. M. (2006). The importance of emotion in psychotherapy approaches. *Journal of Contemporary Psychotherapy, 36*, 59–60.

Smith, D. L. (2003). In W. Dryden (Ed.), *Psychoanalysis in focus*. London: Sage Publications.

Solomon, R. C. (1986). Emotions, Feelings, Contexts. *The Journal of Philosophy, 83*(11), 653–654.

Stern, A. W., Camprodon, J. A., Bermpohl, F., Merabet, L., Rotman, S., Hemond, C., et al. (2007). Shape conveyed by visual-to-auditory sensory substitution activates the lateral occipital complex. *Nature Neuroscience, 10*(6), 687–689.

Strawson, G. (1997). The self. *Journal of Consciousness Studies, 4*(5–6), 405–428.

Strawson, G. (2009). *Selves: An essay in revisionary metaphysics*. Oxford: Clarendon Press.

Stuss, D. T., & Alexander, M. P. (2005). Does damage to the frontal lobes produce impairment in memory? *Current Directions in Psychological Science, 14*(2), 84–88.

Sullivan, P. R. (2006). Are current philosophical theories of consciousness useful to neuroscientists? *Behavior and Philosophy, 34*, 59–70.

Tauber, A. I. (2009). Freud's dreams of reason: The Kantian structure of psychoanalysis. *History of the Human Sciences, 22*(4), 1–29.

Thompson, E. (2001). Empathy and consciousness. *Journal of Consciousness Studies, 8*(5–7), 1–32.

Tirassa, M., Bosco, F. M., & Colle, L. (2006). Rethinking the ontogeny of mindreading. *Consciousness and Cognition, 15*, 197–217.

Tomasello, M., & Rakoczy, H. (2003). What makes human cognition unique. From individual to shared to collective intentionality. *Mind and Language, 8*, 121–147.
Tye, M. (1995). *Ten problems of consciousness: A representational theory of the phenomenal mind*. Cambridge: MIT Press/Bradford Books.
Tye, Q. From Stanford Encyclopedia of Philosophy First published Wed Aug 20, 1997; substantive revision Tue Jul 31, 2007, http://plato.stanford.edu/entries/qualia/. Accessed on 27th October 2011.
Tye, M. (2003). *Consciousness and persons: Unity and identity*. Cambridge: The MIT Press.
Varela, F. J., & Shear, J. (1999a). First-person methodologies: What, why, how? *Journal of Consciousness Studies, 6*(2–3), 1–14.
Varela, F., & Shear, J. (Eds.). (1999b). *The view from within: First person approaches to consciousness*. England: Imprint Academic.
Varela, F., Thompson, E., & Rosch, E. (1991). *The embodied mind: Cognitive science and human experience*. Cambridge: MIT Press.
Vignemonta, F. D. (2007). Habeas corpus: The sense of ownership of one's own body. *Mind and Language, 22*, 427–449.
Vignemonta, F. D., & Fourneretb, P. (2004). The sense of agency: A philosophical and empirical review of the "Who" system. *Consciousness and Cognition, 13*, 1–19.
Washburn, M. (2012). Rethinking the notion of the ego. *Journal of Consciousness Studies, 19*(3–4), 194–222.
Westen, D. (1992). The cognitive self and the psychoanalytic self: Can we put our selves together? *Psychological Inquiry, 3*(1), 1–13.
Wilkes, K. V. (1984). Is consciousness important? *The British Journal for the Philosophy of Science, 35*(3), 223–243.
Wittgenstein, L. (1980). *The blue and brown book*. New York: Harper & Row.
Zahavi, D. (1999). *Self-awareness and alterity: A phenomenological investigation*. Evanston: Northwestern University Press.
Zahavi, D. (2005). *Self and subjectivity: Investigating the first-person perspective*. Cambridge: MIT Press.
Zahavi, D. (2011). Varieties of reflection. *Journal of Consciousness Studies, 18*(2), 9–19.
Zaner, R. M. (1971). *The problem of embodiment: Some contributions to a phenomenology of the body (phaenomenologica)*. Berlin: Springer.
Zarrilli, P. B. (2000). *When the body becomes all eyes: Paradigms, discourses and practices of power in kalarippayattu, a South Indian martial art*. Oxford: Oxford University Press.

Chapter 8
Being and Wellbeing: You, Me and Our Free Will

It is our choices that show what we truly are far more than our capabilities.
—Dumbledore to Harry Potter

J. K. Rowling, *Harry Potter and the Chamber of the Secrets*, 1999, p. 333

Susan Blackmore in an article titled 'She won't be me', in a recent issue of *Journal of Consciousness Studies*, presents two of her theses in a fascinating and provoking manner. The first thesis is that many selves exist, the self by itself is fleeting, and no continuous self exists. And, any of the multitudinous selves or parts of them could inhabit a machine, an information system. The second point she makes, without sufficient reasoned analysis, is that the many selves in the future will be happier and contended, and less depressed, because of the technologies used.

> We might also consider the consequences of the evolution of information in artificial systems and networks. I have suggested that we call the information that is copied, stored, varied and selected by such systems temes (or technological memes, Blackmore, 2010). Temes compete for space and processing capacity within artificial systems just as memes compete for space and processing capacity within human brains. If this is so then we might expect such competition to give rise to all sorts of virtual creatures including experiencing selves.
>
> These selves might be housed in discrete machines such as single computers. In this case they might think of themselves, much as we do, as *being* that machine or inhabiting that machine. But they might not be. They might be distributed among many machines or even exist as relatively stable templates distributed across vast networks. We are a long way from understanding any of this but we might already have an inkling that such creatures might also be fleeting experiencing selves that imagine themselves to be continuing entities when they are not (Blackmore 2012, p. 19) .

There are some significant issues that come up from the above discussion that should worry any researcher in consciousness studies. The existence of selves that are fleeting is not a subject that we can casually discuss limiting them to the futuristic information technology systems. To consider the fleeting self as pieces of information 'copied and stored' in devices is not even a viable postulate for

S. Menon, *Brain, Self and Consciousness*, Studies in Neuroscience, Consciousness and Spirituality, DOI: 10.1007/978-81-322-1581-3_8,

experiments in robotics. The age of the internet and robotics has gone beyond simple information processing tasks and is entering much more complex areas of social media and internet networks that have a viral nature. The self that we should talk about in the context of consciousness has no role to play in the emerging scenario of people-centred information technologies. By adding a concept of self, which is a 'teme', to the artificial systems we will not receive any new insights either about the information systems or about the grand idea of the self that is central to consciousness studies.

8.1 Why the Self is not a 'Teme', and Why I am 'Me'

Our existence even in the moments of awaring discrete events is in the form of an agent and enjoyer of the action not just for that moment but for all moments that preceded and are yet to follow. Such continuity is definitely designed and customized by the culture we come from and the lifestyles we adopt so as to present our personal identities. Yet, there are universal and transcultural factors in experiences that incur from the moments of events. The primary factor that is not of social origin (and perhaps not even biological in origin) is the core-self that provides an unnamed and dislocated space from where the human capacities for coping, hoping and choice-making emerge, particularly when life is at odds. The core-self is not a fleeting self at all and not even a 'thin subject with no ontic depth', as Strawson remarks. According to the materialist position of Strawson, 'a subject of experience is something that exists only if experience exists of which it is the subject'. Since there are many temporary selves, the self as such has no ontic depth and is only a 'cognitively loaded feeling' (Strawson 2009, p. 3).

This essentially means that every experience would have a subject of its own and as experiences appear and disappear the selves also appear and disappear. The central problem in such an argument that takes experience to be the causal agent for the self is that it cannot account for the very existence of experience in the first place. To have a self that experiences the experience at any given moment it is necessary for the subject to have continued from a previous experience. What is that which connects the subject of the previous experience to the subsequent experience? Memories can only give continuity to the content of the experience but not the subject itself since there has to be a prior beholder of memories who can recall them at will. In which case, to whom does the first experience belong? And to whom does the subsequent experience accrue? Experience itself is influenced by the continuity of the experiencer as a continuing self who contributes to the content of each experience with his or her memories, choices, attitudes and responses.

The self is not a point of awareness that exists for a moment, and thus available as many selves. Amazingly, the model of self that is taken by Strawson and many phenomenologists (like Metzinger et al.) and biologists (like Blackmore) is borrowed from information systems, which do not have any metaphysical import. The self they talk about is a linguistic point of reference, and a mode of awareness that ticks away, for a particular event, and which does not exist thereafter. Reminding us of the Humean and Buddhist notions of non-adhering and continuous self, they hold that other than the personal identity marked by culture and society there is no continuous self.

I would think that this is a dangerous and exceedingly superficial view. To deny humans of the organic presence of a continuous self with a core that is not minimal, indiscriminate, fleeting and animalistic, but transcendental at any time will be perhaps not just a casual omission but a serious blunder to commit if one is interested in the character of the person, and deeply philosophical values such as freedom and moral choices. I will not attribute the finer values of human pursuit such as freedom and universal love to a fleeting self that has no say in the course of human life except for discrete events. Nor can these values be attributed to social origin. Of course, our lives and styles as communities customize the expression of these values. But in absolute terms these are values that can only originate from the 'core-self', which is the seat of the body-sense and the self-sense.

Another interesting argument for the nonexistence of a continuous self comes from researchers in affective neuroscience who distinguish between pre-reflective and reflective states of self. A recent position describing the self differently as 'commonsense self' and 'translucent self', which exists only in discrete activities, is as follows:

> This very rarefied high-level self is also exceedingly promiscuous. It flits about and colours whatever experience is currently underway. This translucent self is a movable awareness that emerges in different functional modes, but has no personality *per se*. Where is my real self, for example, when I'm struggling with a Boolean algebra problem? In this case the self seems to 'reside' in the higher neocortical activities of mathematical thinking, but if you suddenly poke me with a pointed stick, then my self will quickly shift to the material body domain. Each new activity—indeed each new moment—brings a new self. If there is such a diaphanous self, then not much can be said about it at this point. One wonders, however, whether we may one day marry the phenomenological self-report of the self-aware subject with sophisticated brain imaging in a way that reveals some unique recursive neural reverberation. We may one day find some neural flash that serves as the material substrate for our familiar sense of translucent subjectivity. This subjectivity is probably an emergent property of various neurochemical systems, some of which reach way down into the limbic and possibly subcortical levels. Below this arid domain of the philosopher's translucent self, however, lies the realm of self that most laypeople contemplate. Here is the self of common sense. A self that has personality—built up over time with beliefs, memories, and life history (Panksepp et al. 2012, pp. 27–28).

To discard the everyday sense of the self as fleeting and commonsense feeling, to attribute rationality to thinking that is not influenced by frail emotions, to enthrone the cognitive capabilities of the self as the attributes of information and robotic systems—these trends have their origins not just in the recent past, but from the ancient times of the Greeks. For instance, the stoics considered absence of emotions, *apatheia*, as a necessary condition for virtue.

The larger question that arises from the disregard for what is fragile and uniquely human as not constituting the essential feature of the human self, is how do we understand the relation between the bland non-being which is proposed and the finer virtues such as freedom and the ultimate goal such as wellbeing. How is the being of the self connected with the incessant and most *passionate* quest for being well in life? What is desire? What is freedom? What is flourishment?

The renewed contemporary interest in values of antiquity such as empathy and compassion, and their biological foundations in mirror neurons and brain-maps, invites us to think about the phasing out of stark divisions between 'me' and the 'other', and to include more of the 'other' in 'me'. This will also bring in studies in cultural neuroscience, social emotions, decision-making, and, most importantly, questions on the self-sense, its peripheries and the ontic core. How much of the self-sense is embodied? Is the self-sense separable from body-schema and its proprioceptive capabilities? What is the role of ownership and agency in binding the self-sense to the body-sense? What is the nature of the self-sense in people with acute impairments in movement and touch senses? Is the self-sense primarily a meaning-making mechanism that overrides bodily limits and disabilities? Signs of self point to the signposts that confirm the existence and workings of the self. To study self is to study the self-sense, its dysfunctions and causes, coping with psychosomatic challenges, feedback mechanisms between the self-sense and the body-sense, and the search for new meanings.

The brain and the self are the final frontiers of consciousness. And it is the boundaries of the brain and the self that we have to continuously contest and expand.

8.2 Values and the Ontological Commitment

Today's mainstream discussion in consciousness studies has brought in the role of the self in an emphatic manner (either to dismiss or affirm it) to understand the workings of the brain. A central question that runs through the major discussions today in neuropsychiatry, phenomenology and philosophy is the place, nature and origin of the self. Self is mostly accepted as an organizing structure, embellishing the lives of an otherwise information processing system with colours, meanings and motivations. Such a tenor also brings together disciplines as disparate as anthropology, cognitive sciences, philosophy and biology.

8.2.1 The Signs of Self

In the recent times, debates on the self have more or less moved away from studying an abstract object to a living subject whose personhood is challenged and framed by neural and mental disposition. Disorders that alter self-perceptions indicate how delicate and thin the neural and mental divide between normalcy and lunacy is. The challenge is not one way, but two ways.[1] We know that the subjective self through experiences, values, attitudes and self-perceptions can alter or influence neural changes to bring in qualitative progress in life.

[1] See Sect. 6.1 in this volume.

Is the self a *subject* for science? In both senses, the response would be 'no'. Self is an 'object' for science, since as a 'subject' it is a non-entity for a scientific discussion. Are we right in perceiving subjectivity and self as objects to be studied in test subjects alone? According to a researcher in neuropsychopharmacology '... it is not only the subjectivity of test subjects, but also that of the neuroscientists themselves, which will be shown to play a crucial role in their experimental practice' (Langlitz 2010, p. 40). Is the sciences' idea of objectivity truly objective?

> Objectivity called for the effacement of the scientific self. This new scientific norm favored mechanical recordings to capture nature with as little human intervention as possible. Self-experimentation became suspect as its results were now regarded as prone to distortion by the scientist's will. Objectivity was born out of a deep-seated distrust, even fear, of the subjective and its inclination to defile an impartial perspective on the world (Langlitz 2010, p. 45).

Traditionally, the self has been included in the domain of religion and philosophy. The interest in science for the self in recent times is in the context of consciousness studies with specific reference to two phenomena exhibited by humans, such as 'altruism' and 'empathy'. Sociobiology has embraced altruism in the context of establishing all behaviours as oriented to selfishness for individual survival. Empathy has entered a relatively new field called neurophenomenology, which looks for the neural processes that underlie empathy.

In our daily life, taking a phenomenological approach to the self, we look for the various dimensions and realms that indicate to us the presence of the self in spite of the difficulties in talking about the self and establishing it with a sound theory. The individual unique stories of our selves are designed by the values and beliefs we cherish, attitudes and perceptions we covertly possess, and memories that run through our thoughts influencing our judgements. With a complex set of personal and interpersonal entities harboured in our selves, in the course of a day, we feel secure at times, insecure at other times, and we constantly search for our notion of wellbeing. A day's activities, we believe, have the purpose of leading us to a being-well state, or in biological terms, to a steady flow of dopamine in our blood stream.

8.3 The Being-Well Agenda

The central motivation for understanding the brain, the self and through these two, consciousness, is to rediscover human wellbeing especially for a person who is challenged by mental conflicts and other dissipative disorders. Along with other disciplines, psychology too is shifting its focus of study from a pathological orientation to a positive orientation of life. What the study of pathological states finally seeks is rediscovery of states of happiness and positive adaptation.

The primary distinction between pleasure and happiness (wellbeing) is that the first borrows a significant amount of content from sensations, and the latter is a deeper state that is situated in an undefined core-self. While pleasure is dependent on objects, people and situations, wellbeing is dependent on the inner disposition of the individual, his or her sense of autonomy, virtues and passion for common good.

Wellbeing mostly is experienced in our lives when we find a meaning and purpose to living. Wellbeing which lasts long and is eudaemonic, is dependent not on one factor but several factors (Diener 1984) and evokes a sense of meaning that is derived from pursuing goals in the service of something of wider significance than oneself (Seligman 2002). Eudaemonic wellbeing is also different from short-term pleasures in being multidimensional. An eudaemonically happy person will exhibit autonomy, environmental mastery, self-acceptance, positive relations with others, personal growth and purpose in life (Ryff 1989). Biological markers of health are correlated with eudaemonic wellbeing and not with short-term pleasures (Ryff et al. 2004).

Multidisciplinary studies defining the being-well agenda are also unanimous that wellbeing, or lasting happiness, is not only the ultimate life goal but also a means to pursue other goals, and is responsible for life satisfaction. Subjective wellbeing is often interpreted to mean experiencing a high level of positive affect, a low level of negative affect, and a high degree of satisfaction with one's life (Deci and Ryan 2008).

In almost all of wellbeing studies, the two life traits that clearly emerge are 'meaning' and 'purpose'. Can meaning be achieved through narratives, the stories of our life that we continuously write in our mind? The tradition of narratives, termed 'meaningful stories' by Saks (1999), attempts to smoothen the uneven edges of mental life and find renewed meanings in life and living. The narrative account of life stories gives an emotional closure to the conflict experienced and a new beginning to renewed living.

There are two positions on the causation and placement of meaning: one focus is the person and the other the society. Personal meaning emerges by the self-organization and explication of one's own emotional experience; and optimal adaptation involves an integration of reason and emotion (Greenberg 2002, p. 87). The alternate view is that meaning does not inhere in the individual or in objects, but is, instead, social. Knowing what objects (self, others, relationships, and communities) mean to people illuminates how social actors live out the often unequal patterns and arrangements that we call 'society' (Fields, Copp and Kleinman 2007, p. 164).

Whatever the source of origin is, we do have a need to knit together disparate edges, find new meanings, give up old beliefs, form new beliefs, and through all these rest our self in its core space. Three concepts central to James' (1985; first published in 1902) thinking, which endorse the resting of the self, are 'healthy-mindedness', 'happiness' and saintliness that he develops in his lectures on *The Religion of Healthy-mindedness*, *The Sick Soul* and *Saintliness.* According to James, mind cure is possible by '··· relaxing, letting go, ··· giving your little private convulsive self a rest, and finding that a greater Self is there' (p. 111). What is certain is, '··· that we can experience union with *something* larger than ourselves and in that union find our greatest peace' (p. 525). According to James, such a cure for the mind might undermine the scientific method, but its successes can be verified experimentally.

Is neuroscience correct in conjecturing that altruism is the only behaviour to favour individual survival, and that choice-making is an epiphenomenon of neural processes? Is our belief in free will and agency of action a chimera in neural terms? Perhaps we have to consider a complex vocabulary such as perception, motives, intentions, sense of agency, meaning, commitment, purpose, reasoning, rationality, etc., while discussing accounts of action (Bruun and Langlais 2003, p. 40).

8.3.1 Inner Narratives and Moral Agency

It is a widespread assumption that the brain initiates action even before we make conscious choices, following the works of Libet (1993), and hence freedom of choice is a wrong or illusory feeling that we humans have. Ralph Ellis gives a detailed and telling response to such a view:

> Libet et al. show that a readiness potential in the supplementary motor area precedes the conscious experience of choice, so that when we experience ourselves as choosing to do an action the brain actually has already initiated the action. This finding that a Readiness Potential precedes consciousness of action decisions is quickly interpreted by some philosophers to mean choice is illusory. But this conclusion is not supported by a fuller neuroscientific look at how the brain works… The RP indicates that the action command has been initiated, in order to form an action image, but not that it has been disinhibited. When we 'choose' to do the action, we disinhibit the command—corresponding to Libet's 'veto power'. The 'veto power' is not an exceptional occurrence, but accompanies every willed action. When we choose not to 'veto' (disinhibit) an action command, we experience ourselves simply as deciding once and for all to do the action that the initial RP imaged. … The choice not to 'veto' that action is not a separate experience from the choice to do the action. Instead, the subjective feeling of deciding to do the action (having already imaged ourselves doing it) correlates with the disinhibition of the command. The point at which we disinhibit the command is the point at which we experience ourselves as deciding to go through with the action (Ellis 2005, p. 145–147).

Has ethics a reason to fear from neuroscience? If moral agency and deeper desires to genuinely help, support and care the other person, are a figment of the brain, then can deeply humane issues such as wellbeing and self-transformation be accounted for? Ellis continues with his theory of meta-emotion and effective imagery:

> … Ethics has nothing to fear from neuroscience, even if the latter is completely deterministic. Moral agency requires the ability to use self-generated imagery to trigger the appropriate feelings in our selves, based on a desire to act morally… The rational capacity of the prefrontal cortex allows humans both to generalize a universal altruism from the natural mammalian feelings of altruism toward certain specific individuals; and also to generate imagery or narratives at will, even where the imagery or narrative is to be used to trigger feelings that we do not yet have, but believe we should have. In the case of morally useful feelings that we would like to have, the use of imagery to trigger the feeling is motivated by the feeling of universalized altruism, which makes us want to do what is best on the whole… (Ellis 2005, p. 152).

Our plights are often due to an overactive and reactive sympathetic nervous system which has been used to only the stressful choice of either fight or flight. The only way to quieten the conflicted system is to bring in the qualities of calmness and stability, and to arouse the parasympathetic system, which is responsible for the resting of the system. The resting of the self, tired by its myriad experiences, in its core for some is a once-in-a-while activity through soul searching, and for others this is a continuous disposition. The *Bhagavad Gita*, for instance, describes the supreme state of *Samadhi* as a continuous rest of the self, even while engaged in physical and mental activities, in non-individuated consciousness.[2] If such a resting place is not constantly invoked we see a struggling self with its boundaries shifting not only because of neural features but also with the challenges received from emotional upsurges, personal insecurities and social living. The hidden possibilities of the core-self are revealed, according to an Upanishadic text, when the inward-looking eye is favoured.

The closest scholarly practice in formulating theories on consciousness that emphasizes an engaged perspective falls in the field of folk psychology. Character virtues, moral principles, optimism and positive emotions, are found to increase resilience, coping with adverse situations and prosocial behaviour. Not much of serious discussions on consciousness take cues from the content of our inner lives and folk psychology. This is one reason that we continue to have disengaged discussions on ethics and morality without having to bring their practice in our lives as an imperative for understanding them. In addition, we discuss consciousness as an information processing system whose best model is a computational mind.

What we tend to ignore is that the content of our folk psychology and inner narratives play a central role in adjudicating our attitudes towards events that happen around us. The non-emotional, discrete, cognitive agent that we try to model through artificial systems is not the one who is housed in the private centre of our life. The agent of action and the owner of experience that inheres in us is an engaged, complex person with biases and perspectives that are neither neutral nor person-detached. First-person centrality is not a detached perspective about the content of another person's experience, but is an engaged perspective with the coloured content of one's inner life. As Shoemaker states:

> I certainly think that it is essential to a philosophical understanding of the mental that we appreciate that there is a first person perspective on it, a distinctive way mental states present themselves to the subjects whose states they are, and that an essential part of the philosophical task is to give an account of mind which makes intelligible the perspective mental subjects have on their own mental lives.
>
> … There are a number of areas in the philosophy of mind in which first-person imaginings have played an important role in philosophical reflection. These include the issue of whether the identity over time of a person involves the identity of a body or brain, the issue of whether disembodied existence of persons is a possibility, the issue of whether 'spectrum inversion' is a possibility, and the issue of whether mental states can be identical with physical states of bodies or with functional states realized in physical states of bodies. In many of these cases I agree with the possibility claims that first-person imaginings have been used to support. I think that personal identity does not require bodily identity or brain identity, and I think that spectrum inversion is a possibility (Shoemaker 1994, p. 7–8).

---

[2] *Bhagavad Gita*, 4: 24.

Disciplines such as neuroscience and neuropsychology will influence the understanding of other minds and our own in a substantial manner in the years to come. Brain, self and consciousness will continue to be objects of natural kind for the sciences.

Contributions from brain studies have today changed the way we address several problems that required complex and challenging answers a decade or two back. Consciousness has unarguably become the most charming contender to walk the ramp for not just one but many allied disciplines that border neuroscience, cognitive psychology, neuropsychiatry, neurophilosophy, and even biogenetics. Some say that the one area that will emerge in the coming years as the most important in the history of humankind is 'neuronomics'—the nexus between insights from neuroscience, and the philosophy and psychology of choice-making abilities.

Another area where the issue of agency is central, but not discussed enough, is that of spiritual experiences. The meaning of human identity is certainly going to be debated in a manner that has never occurred before. The challenge to re-humanize, re-emotionalize and de-commodity the person will persist as long as there is an unsaid and unarticulated desire to reach and experience the finer realms of consciousness. Such a challenge will also occasionally revert to the reflexive and skeptical question of the possibility and veracity in a brain studying another brain, or consciousness understanding another consciousness. Is consciousness fundamentally evasive to an observer-observed paradigm? Is consciousness translucent to a knower and an agent?

The experience of agency is most significant not only in the formation of a first-person perspective, but also in the development of social cognition, inter-subjective values, such as empathy, and coexistence. The possibility of transformation and transcendence in human experiences continuously remind us yet another significant dimension of human consciousness namely spiritual experience (Menon and Bodhananda 2003) and its relation to agency. An exciting enquiry would be to explore how the 'integrality' provided by agency and the effacement of selfhood in spiritual experience, could be correlated.

The evading characteristic of consciousness makes it more appealing to almost all disciplines, including good old philosophy. But the fact of the matter is that even to have some minimalistic idea of what consciousness is, a whole set of parameters have to be factored in. The major challenge is to understand ways by which the personal experience and the impersonal brain are connected. Such a challenge will also lead us to discover routes to positive and transformative living.

8.4 Desire and the Self

A fundamental factor necessary in tracing the boundary of the self is the sense of security we live with. The sense of security is constituted by: (1) the fears that decide biases in responding to situations, and (2) the nature of desire and its goal.

Just as we have a sense of our body and a sense of our self, the sense of security that is deeply engrained is fundamental to our physical and psychological equilibrium. Often, we are oblivious to the subtle existence of such a sense playing a crucial role in our decision-making activities. Fear, desire and their goal are invariably related to our sense of security. Here, once again, what we refer to is not just the quantified amount of security (health, nuclear, etc.) based on probabilities and statistical data, but the subliminal sense of security that the self seeks. All our actions, responses and meaning seeking are founded on the sense of security that we feel in our selves often in a nonverbalized and covert manner.

Philosophically or otherwise there is agreement that it is desire which invokes action with the help of intention. Desires produce intentions, and intentions lead to actions. Desire refers to having an urge for something, the need to possess or dispossess, the intention to achieve. On the one hand, cognitive elements constitute desires; on the other, desires are imbued with emotions, values and world views. The psychology of desire is a subject that has brought in controversial theories of the unconscious and personality traits..

What causes a desire? What is achieved through the fulfilment (or non-fulfilment) of the desire? How does desire and its ultimate purpose of eudaemonic wellbeing, or common good, influence our biases in perceiving purpose? How objective are we in considering the merits and adverse outcomes without downplaying or exaggerating either? How do the biases interfere in decision-making process?

The last two questions are significant particularly when studies have shown that when making choices and solving problems of complexity, rational elements are found missing and we are influenced by 'a-rational' factors. 'People do not typically solve problems, make decisions or reach conclusions using the kind of standard, conscious and rational processes that they were more or less assumed to be using.... When people were observed making choices and solving problems of interesting complexity, the rational and the logical elements were often missing' (Reber 1993, p. 13). Such a revelation brings back to us the flaw in the idea of emotions lacking cognitive content.

Desire motivates action. And the sense of security decides the emergence of desires. Our responses are dependent on our sense of security, which in turn is driven by fear and anxiety. It is established theory that while fear and anxiety, to a certain extent, perform functions evolutionarily engraved by our biology (fight or flight), they also create health hazards when taken out of proportion. Fear of the unknown is a psychological force that overrides any rational and quantified account of possible threats and adverse outcomes. Subjective identity is defined by the fear of the unknown.

Let us look at some phenomenological content:

1. I said something hurtful to A, because of which I do not know what might A's response would be in the near and long-term future.

Did I say something wrong?

What are the consequences and relevance for me?

2. I desired for something. And have engaged in relevant action leading to its fulfilment.

Did I put myself in an unknown space in the course of my action?
Was my desire legitimate?
Can I analyse my actions and reason for that particular desire objectively?
Am I in control?
What are the fundamental mental forces behind these motivations?

1. Desire for something which is yet to be achieved,
2. Inability to gauge (long-term) consequences, and,
3. Anxiety and discomfort.

Are human actions, in general, free of these three fundamental mental forces? Can we be free of desires?

We wish to control outcomes. But do we have control on the multiple factors that decide the outcomes?

In fact, we could say that, no action can be performed without the motivation that springs from desire. No amount of consequential thinking and conceptual tools will give as an exhaustive scale of outcomes. And, no action is free from some amount of expectation. All actions are founded in desire; anticipation of outcomes, and some degree of anxiety. These three subliminal psychological forces together determine our *sense* of security.

The sense of security is the sense we have of displacement (or its absence); of losing (or not); and being (or not) in control. As individuals, and unique individuals with our makings determined by a host of private factors which are psychological and cultural, we perceive danger and displacement determined by our sense of security. An optimal sense of security is decided by the nature of choices and decision-making, and also our tolerance to outcomes.

Are our choices well-informed? Are the subliminal forces behind the nature of choice brought to the light of conscious analysis? Do we address the 'what if' question (for example, what if something goes wrong)? Do we make better decisions when there are more choices? Sheena Iyengar writes: 'Perhaps it is not that people are made unhappy by the decisions they make in the face of abundant options but that they are instead unsure—that they are burdened by the responsibility of distinguishing good from bad decisions' (Iyengar 2000, p. 1004).

While receiving options and making choices from the many available, our minds convert the objects we see to symbols. For instance when I am given a range of soda drinks, though the content of all are the same, the one (or none) I would opt for is decided by the symbolic value I give for it. Often when we see objects, we then convert them to symbols so that we can make decisions in tune with our perceptions and beliefs. Our biases are tuned either by the apparent package of the object or its deeper content. This is because, in spite of our respective disciplinary training and professions, we have private minds and personal lives to lead. Our objective and rational thinking are subjected to the vagaries (or richness) of a subjective, personal mind. However much we dismiss our selves as fleeting, the decisions that we make, the desires and biases that we possess, the will to influence our being, wellbeing, arise from a private self and are directed by our choice-making

Richard Restak discusses the impossibility of neural events to address our acts of free will, though he conjectures that language could be behind the expressions of human motivation.

> What brain events correspond with conscious experience? For instance, what is going on in my brain when, in a restaurant, I order a chocolate soufflé? How does it differ from events that would accompany my choosing apple pie à la mode instead? Implicit in such questions is the assumption that there must exist correlations between my choices and the events going on in my brain. But what are they? The answer immediately introduces two levels of discourse masquerading as only one. To choose a chocolate soufflé is an act of will. It requires the use of words in a language that will be meaningful to the waiter and involves innumerable variables that can never be reduced to an explanation at the level of a chemical slipping across a synapse. Why am I in the restaurant in the first place? What does my ordering of a highly caloric dessert imply about my attitude toward obesity? To ask such questions is immediately to participate in a long-standing debate regarding the place of language in human motivation (Restak 1982, pp. 102–103).

The interrelations between being and wellbeing up two questions that are phenomenological and metaphysical at the same time. These questions are, 'What is consciousness from what standpoint?', and 'Who is asking?' The first question emphasizes the category of definition, and the second factors the analyst not only as an objective, detached thinker but also as an involved participant in the understanding of 'consciousness'. The complexity of the being of the subject is such that every factor employed in the understanding of the phenomenon opens to further leads in defining it. The mystery of consciousness is that there is an organic process of the experiencer, 'the conscious being' integrating the knowledge about itself into its beingness. There is a tension between 'the experiencer' and 'the experienced', which exists not only as a theoretical obstruct but also as an ontological challenge. And it is this tension which emphasizes the connections between the being and wellbeing aspects of the self.

From the Eastern traditions, the spatial model that is presented by Patanjali, the master of the yogic traditions, attempts to understand the uncanny intertwining between emotions and cognitive content in knowing. His yoga psychology is woven around the discussion of five mental planes (*citta bhumi*), five cognitive modes (*citta vrtti*), nine mental afflictions (*antaraya*), and five causes of pain (*citta klesa*). The concept of *citta klesa*, in particular, is rooted in whole and organic experience. Patanjali enumerates five causes of pain—*avidya* (ignorance), *asmita* (I-sense), *raga* (like), *dvesa* (dislike), *abhinivesa* (attachment to body and life). What is interesting here is that the nature of these five causes is not wholly mental but also shares attributes that concerns the person as an individual with lived experiences. It relates to existential and ontological pains. Afflictions arise from the person as a whole. What is pivotal in this model is that the centre of discussion is not emotion as a discrete affect entity. The complex states of the mind are given focus, from the context of which cognition, conation and affect are discussed (Menon 2009).

8.5 Self, Character and Wellbeing

The recent trends in neuroscience support a self that has no abiding existence. The central challenge that the 'fleeting self' or 'no self' theorists have to address is how we account for character and moral agency of the person. Memories or a changing identity that are based on context and culture do help in understanding the fleeting self but do not account for the existence of free will and responsibility. Character cannot be imagined to be belonging to a person who has no self, or a fleeting self. So, are we saying that moral agency and free will have to be understood as special kind of virtues that cannot be explained adequately with the help of a culture of fleeting behaviours and changing perceptions of the person?

The ideas about free will, character and the self are to be seen in a common space if we have to appreciate that the human consciousness possess deeper levels of reflective capability and the ability to relate to an undefined core-self at the time of challenges to the physical and mental aspects of one's identity. Behaviours are expressions of one's character nourished by the virtues that is treasured. One's sense of freedom to make choices without being biased by favourable or unfavourable outcomes indicates that the human mind is not a vacant tablet and the self is not a product of language and changing environment.

The major debate about the existence of free will, and the presence of unconscious acts directed by the brain, focuses on our bodily behaviours and its unpredictable outcomes. Even if there is a biological disposition for our bodies to act without the meta-awareness of a decision already taken by the bio-psychological apparatus of the brain that do not amount to propose the absence of an abiding self. To defend the availability of free will, we will have to move away from the body and brain based arguments that are directed by the neural behaviour and focus on the idea of the core-self which is also the source for invoking self-transformation. The discussion on character and moral agency cannot be fairly placed in the context of neural behaviour but only in the possibility of character for a continuing self in spite of changes in the person's biology, environment and culture.

> All of us will find ourselves repeatedly placed in situations that we cannot entirely control and acted upon by forces that we cannot control. Character has a vital role in how we act. That is, to have a character is to act in such a way that the person one is plays a major role in any explanation of one's behavior. To have no character is to act in such a way that one's behavior might be viewed as (at least approximately) the product of forces acting on one. Thus, the person who always yields to temptation quickly, without a struggle, would be spoken of as having no character, as would the extreme conformist who always does what is expected of him or her (Kupperman 1991, p. 7).

In order to connect the self and one's character, one's experience of free will, and perception of responsibility, it is essential to envision the self which abides and integrates the changes. The nihilism and relativism about the concept of the self almost misses the ontology of the self that is ever-present even with an anarchist and a critic of the core-self.

> Admittedly, assigning someone a definite character of some sort does not preclude change, but to have a character does require a degree of stability, which perhaps never can be guaranteed. Is talk of character a way of papering over variations, fluctuations, and so forth? Does it (as might be asked also of the traditional stable, enduring self) represent more the simple expression of a wish, and a requirement we impose on life, than a reality? (Kupperman 1999, p. 60).

8.5.1 Meaning and Purpose

Another crucial factor that is ignored is the importance of narratives that we form for ourselves and others in our lives. Whether we succeed or fail, we have an incessant need to make meaning out of discrete life events and life as a continuum. Kupperman comments that the importance of a strong character can be seen if we reflect on what it is for a life to have, or to lack, a meaning. Further, to have a meaningful life, 'is to have a life that lends itself to being made into a story: A life not only in which there are interesting things, but also in which there are connections so that parts of the life assume significance in relation to other parts' (Kupperman 1991, p. 135).

The inner need to discover and experience meaning influences our ability to formulate purposes and make attempts to achieve them. A fleeting self at least in an apparent sense gives the impression of a casual perception or disregard for any kind of permanence. Since a fleeting self cannot believe in permanence, as a consequence see others' selves too as fleeting and without the interest in long-lasting and life-changing values. In short, our being and its character are interconnected with our wellbeing. A fleeting self can desire for changing degrees of pleasures that is governed by other changing objects and causes. It is a permanent self that hopes and believes in happiness that is not dependent on changing external agents and objects but that which is invoked from an unknown space of the core-self. Hence, the stark distinction between hedonistic joy and the common good shared by eudaemonic wellbeing. The notion of hedonistic joy and the fleeting self theory follow a social science model, and the eudaemonic wellbeing model follows the theory of the already existent which is unravelled. Deci and Ryan write:

> The hedonic approach uses … the standard social science model, which considers the human organism initially to be relatively empty and thus malleable, such that it gains its meaning in accord with social and cultural teachings. In contrast, the Eudemonic approach ascribes content to human nature and works to uncover that content and to understand the conditions that facilitate versus diminish it (Deci and Ryan 2008, p. 3).

Eudaemonic wellbeing requires acts that follow virtues and an exercise of free will and responsibility. Without a self that has content gained from previous experiences and guided by the undefined space of the core-self, the attainment of eudaemonia is impossible. In effect, eudaemonic wellbeing rests on the invoking of the core space which is also the home for values, freedom and the sense of autonomy that encourages choice-making.

References

Blackmore, S. (2012). She won't be me. *Journal of Consciousness Studies, 19*(1–2), 16–19.
Bruun, H., & Langlais, R. (2003). On the embodied nature of action. *Acta Sociologica, 46*(1), 31–49.
Deci, E. L., & Ryan, R. M. (2008). Hedonia, Eudaimonia, and well-being: An introduction. *Journal of Happiness Studies, 9*, 1–11.
Diener, E. (1984). Subjective well-being. *Psychological Bulletin, 95*, 542–575.
Ellis, R. D. (2005). The roles of imagery and meta-emotion in deliberate choice and moral psychology. *Journal of Consciousness Studies, 12*(8–10), 140–157. G. Colombetti, & E. Thompson, (Eds.).
Fields, J., Copp, M., & Kleinman, S. (2007). Symbolic interactionism, inequality and emotions. In J. E. Stets, & J. H. Turner (Eds.), *Handbook of the sociology of emotions* (pp. 155–178). Springer Science.
Greenberg, L. (2002). Emotion-focused therapy: Coaching clients to work through feelings. Washington: American Psychological Association.
Harnad (2005). *The New York Book Review.*
Iyengar, S. S. (2000). When choice is demotivating: Can one desire too much of a good thing? *Journal of Personality and Social Psychology, 79*(6), 1004.
James, W. (1985). *The varieties of religious experience: edited with an introduction.* In: M. E. Marty (Ed.) New York: Penguin Classics.
Kupperman, J. J. (1991). *Character*. Oxford: Oxford University Press.
Kupperman, J. J. (1999). *Learning from Asian philosophy*. Oxford: Oxford University Press.
Langlitz, N. (2010). The persistence of the subjective in neuropsychopharmacology: observations of contemporary hallucinogen research. *History of the Human Sciences, 23*(1), 37–57.
Libet, B. (1993). *Neurophysiology of Consciousness: Selected papers and new essays*. Boston: Birkhäuser
Menon, S. (2009). The rain clouds of mind-modifications and the shower of transcendence: Yoga and Samadhi in Patanjali yoga sutra. In R. Rao (Ed.), *Yoga and parapsychology: Empirical research and theoretical essays* (pp. 169–199). Delhi: Motilal Banarsidass.
Menon, S., & Bodhananda, S. (2003). *Dialogues: philosopher meets seer*. New Delhi: BlueJay Books.
Panksepp, J., Asma, S., Curran, G., Gabriel, R., & Greif, T. (2012). The philosophical implications of affective neuroscience. *Journal of Consciousness Studies, 19*(3–4), 6–48.
Petranker, J. (2003). Inhabiting conscious experience: Engaged objectivity in the first-person study of consciousness. *Journal of Consciousness Studies, 10*(12), 3–23.
Reber, A. S. (1993). *Implicit learning and tacit knowledge: An essay on the cognitive unconscious*. New York: Oxford University Press.
Restak, R. M. (1982). The archaeology of the self. *The Wilson Quarterly, 6*(3), 98–104.
Ryff, C. D. (1989). Happiness is everything, or is it? Explorations on the meaning of psychological well-being. *Journal of Personality and Social Psychology, 57*, 1069–1081.
Ryff, C., Singer, B., & Love, G. (2004). Positive health: Connecting well-being with biology. *Philoosphical Transactions*, 1383–1394.
Saks, E. R. (1999). *Interpreting interpretation: The limits of hermeneutic psychoanalysis*. New Haven: Yale University Press.
Seligman, M. (2002). *Authentic happiness*. New York: Free Press.
Shoemaker, S. (1994). The first-person perspective. *Proceedings and Addresses of the American Philosophical Association, 68* (2), 7–22.
Strawson, G. (2009). *Selves: An essay in revisionary metaphysics*. Oxford: Clarendon Press.

Chapter 9
Beyond the Brain: The Final Frontiers of Consciousness

> *Two friendly birds sit on the same tree; One jumps up and down pecking at sour and sweet fruits;*
> *The other silently observes, without eating.*
>
> —Mundaka Upanishad, 3.1.1.

We might conjecture that the journey into the unchartered space of consciousness began since the dawn of human life, or since the use of language, or since the advent of disciplines such as biology, philosophy and psychology, or since we became curious to know the brain better. How far have we reached, and how much distance have we covered in this journey?

We, mostly following the falsifiability principle, have gained new wisdom and discarded old ideas on complex concepts that relate to the biological organ that is the brain, and the psychological organ that is the mind. In this route we have also understood that the self whether we call it synaptic, or the neocortical, or the unconscious, or the spiritual, is the inescapable presence that gives meaning to the coexistence of the mind and the brain.

Without the self, there is no purpose for the existence of the brain and the mind. We cannot legitimize our enquiry without a self to experience, a self to discover the unchartered spaces of consciousness. Essentially, the traveller in the sojourn of consciousness is the self itself. The self brings to us the mystery of consciousness, its origin and nature, by pointing to the limits of the physical and psychological structures that we know through the brain and the mind.

The major puzzle that consciousness presents to us is in finding the evading agent and the enjoyer in and through the experience. We use brain imaging techniques, encephalographs, radioactive tracer dyes, clinical diagnostic tests, cognitive and AI experiments to trace the contours of the agent of action and the enjoyer of experience, knowing well the possibilities and limits of methodologies.

Richard Restak writes:

> Can the brain understand itself? There is no way for us to stand back and 'objectively observe' the brain or even theorize about it, without encountering constraints that are

S. Menon, *Brain, Self and Consciousness*, Studies in Neuroscience, Consciousness and Spirituality, DOI: 10.1007/978-81-322-1581-3_9,

> inherent in our neuronal networks. To what extent can 'reality' or 'truth' be ascertained when the inquiring organ—the brain—itself exhibits significant perceptual biases that can never be altered? (Restak 1982, p. 104).

The crux of the puzzle that consciousness carries with it inspires us to conceptualize ways in which the brain and the self mutually challenge each other. Consciousness is fringed by neural and self-attributes.

As we know today, the brain is not an isolated biological organ, but a *self-challenged brain*, by its very existence and sustenance. Conversely, we concur that the self cannot be a completely abstract entity that reveals only through experience, but is to be seen as a *brain-challenged self*. Hence, better methodologies to understand consciousness will have to emerge from positing the brain-challenged self and the self-challenged brain as the heart of the problem, and not viewing the brain and the self in isolation. Without the brain we may not have the cognitive capacities to enquire into the intricacies of biological complexity that influence the sophisticated existence of life. Without the self, there is no joy in enquiring into the most challenging and unpredictable organ of the body. It is the self which gives us what we humanly call 'fun' and 'joy'.

The final frontiers of consciousness are the brain and the self. The self concretizes the 'harder problem' of consciousness. In this journey to see and be in the unchartered space, theories might fail, but experiences will give new insights.

The *self-in-the-brain* and *brain-in-the-self* might also require us to see the brain not just in the vat and the self not just in culture. The abstract possibilities of the unknown self surprise us experientially and therapeutically beyond the confines of culture and biology. The brain and the self are cross-wired in a fashion that the challenges between these two decide the course we take to locate consciousness. In the process, we concede with the biological imperativeness of an evolving brain and an emergent self. The greatest challenge before consciousness studies is to ask and then to proceed to chart clear pathways that begin with the physicality of neural structures and end with the subjectivity of the experience, though it is a near to impossible task. With that challenge also arise questions such as:

Is the brain hard-wired for each sensation separately and without change?

What is the nature of the intervention of the conscious agent and its role in building adaptability?

What is the role of memory as the bridge builder between physicality (of the brain) and subjectivity (of the self)?

How do the brain and the self together create the conspiracy of experience where the physicality of the brain is lost in the subjectivity of the self?

How can we conceptualize the self as the meaning-giver having both emergent and abiding features?

Primarily, is the self the highway to the space of consciousness?

9.1 Normality of Self and Alternate Self-experiences

Experiments on plotting neural correlates of mystical experiences are just about a decade old. Commenced by the initial work of Newberg et al. (2001), and others, and with the advent of sophisticated brain sensing machines such as fMRI (functional magnetic resonance imaging), and SPECT (single photon emission computed tomography), certain experiences termed 'mystical' are being increasingly addressed by neuroscientists. This new approach to study mystical experiences is called 'spiritual neuroscience', which like other branches of neuroscience considers mystical experiences as well to be mediated by the brain.

> The turn of the new millennium has seen the emergence of 'Spiritual neuroscience', a field of scientific investigation at the crossroads of psychology, religion and spirituality, and neuroscience. The main objective of this novel domain of research is to explore the neural underpinnings of religious/spiritual/mystical experiences (RSMEs). ... One of the basic assumptions of spiritual neuroscience is that RSMEs are brain-mediated, as are all other aspects of human experience. With respect to this issue, it is of paramount importance to fully appreciate that elucidating the neural substrates of these experiences does not diminish or depreciate their meaning and value, and that the external reality of 'God' can neither be confirmed nor disconfirmed by delineating the neural correlates of RSMEs (Beauregard and Paquette 2006, p. 186).

Two of the prominent studies locate the temporal lobe, orbitofrontal cortex, and the parietal cortex to be the source for the microseizures that are responsible for the experience of mystical experiences in Carmelite nuns (Beauregard and Paquette 2006) and Franciscan nuns (Newberg et al. 2001). The alterations in the body-schema felt during mystical experiences are, according to these studies, the resultant of the involvement of several brain regions and systems. According to Newberg (2001, p. 53) '... if God does indeed exist, the only place he can manifest his existence would be in the tangled neural pathways and physiological structures of the brain'.

Recent studies on the connections (structural and ontological) between the brain and god have brought in a humanizing picture of the brain. These works do not move away from the fundamental (scientific) position that however profound the god experience is, it will have to be channelled and experienced through the brain. The major hypotheses that underlie these works are the role of the association areas of the brain, myths that underlie the concept of religious belief, integral function of the sympathetic and parasympathetic nervous system, and the brain's capacity to distinguish between the self and the rest (not-self) outside it, and also to alter or extend this division.

Newberg's studies on the neural correlates of meditative experiences of Tibetan monks have particularly shown change in all the association areas and, in particular, less activity in the orientation association area or the pre-frontal cortex. It is to be also said that these studies, with amazing details of the human capacity to form a self and to continuously extend its limits, have been made possible by the advancement in brain scanning technologies. The most significant technologies being single positron emission computed tomography (SPECT), different forms of positron emission tomography (PET), low-resolution electromagnetic tomography (LORETA), electroencephalography (EEG) and quantitative electroencephalography (QEEG).

A widespread, if not mainstream, theory following Newberg et al. is about the physicalist version of religious and mystical experiences, that they have a neural location. Many researchers consider that religious and mystical experiences are processed in the temporal lobe and limbic system. Inspired by this theory often religious and meditational experiences are translocated (from the natural environs of the Tibetan monk or the Franciscan nun) to lab conditions where such experiences are triggered, watched, and even controlled. One of the emergent hypotheses from such experiments is that similar experiences can be induced in normal brains with the help of electrical stimulation of the specific brain areas, by administering psychedelic substances, or is available as a natural experience for a patient with temporal epilepsy.

Saver and Rabin write:

> Religious experience is brain-based. This should be taken as an unexceptional claim. All human experience is brain-based, including scientific reasoning, mathematical deduction, moral judgment, and artistic creation, as well as religious states of mind. Determining the neural substrates of these states does not automatically lessen or demean their spiritual significance. The external reality of religious percepts is neither confirmed nor disconfirmed by establishing brain correlates of religious experience. Indeed, it has been argued that demonstrating the existence of a neural apparatus sustaining religious experience can reinforce belief because it provides evidence that a higher power has so constructed humans as to possess the capacity to experience the divine (Saver and Rabin 1997, p. 498).

The most important question to sceptics as well as experiences is: is religious or mystical experience always correlated to some form of brain anomaly or dysfunction? Is it true to pinpoint religious experience to aberrations in the temporal lobe? How sensitive it is to the history of religious experiences to qualify the limbic system as the 'primary substrate' (Saver and Rabin 1997) of religious experience?

Perhaps, we could consider one of the strong arguments against the 'neural correlate of religious experience' approach in the idea expressed by Michael Kozart, a doctor at the UCLA Neuropsychiatric Institute, Center for the Health Sciences in Los Angeles, in response to Saver and Rabin's article. Favouring the theory of 'socially distributed belief system', he writes:

> The weakness of this article stems from the fact that no adequate formulation of religious phenomena is provided. What the authors suggest is that 'the direct sensory awareness of God or the divine…is a quintessential mark of specifically religious experience' (p. 499). However, a quick review of world religions demonstrates that the concept of God or divinity is by no means ubiquitous, and therefore by no means quintessential for religious experience… the quintessential mark of specifically religious experience cannot be related to the direct sensory awareness of God but rather is related to membership within a socially distributed belief system. We ought not presume that states of altered temporolimbic activity account for genuine religious experience. Such states account for, say, temporolimbic epilepsy—not religious experience. The clinical phenomenology of temporolimbic epilepsy may well be mediated through

> culturally constructed religious symbols (say God), but we ought not confuse those symbols with the original context from which they were derived (genuine religious experience).In making this mistake, we risk impoverishing the essential meaning of religion (Kozart 1998).

The history of mind studies has greatly favoured naturalistic interpretations, in order to compare with something structurally closer. But then by this approach do we undermine a phenomenon uniquely central for the human experience in order to favour a comparable other in the natural world? Edward Kelly and Emily Kelly write:

> Our a priori commitment to a conventional physicalist account of the mind has rendered us systematically incapable of dealing adequately with the mind's most central properties. We need to rethink that commitment (Kelly et al. 2007, p. 42).

In recent discussions, the debate has moved from the existence (or non-existence) of God to the representation of God experience in the brain. The first debate perhaps is a philosophical whirlpool. But the second opens up possibilities of dialogue on not just the nature of religious experience but also the myriad baseline and alternate human experiences. Along with the second debate comes the re-entry of myths and cultural expressions to understand mystical experience from an evolutionary standpoint.

Studies conducted by Newberg and d'Aquili carve a different space amongst the increasing number of brain theories of mystical and religious experience. Their works (d'Aquili and Newberg 1993; Newberg et al. 2001) are notable for ideas that do not claim a strict, naturalistic interpretation. To list some: they claim that the association areas of brain play a greater role in mystical experiences; they term neurological anchors of mind 'cognitive operators' and 'cognitive imperative'; state that myths are larger frameworks to understand alternate experiences; that deafferentation of left orientation area causes complete loss of the sense of self.

Newberg and d'Aquili suggest a continuum that ranges between the experience of baseline reality and profound unitary consciousness (absolute, unitary being). The absolute, unitary being experience is marked by clear neural signs such as increased blood flow to the pre-frontal cortex which is the area of concentration and decreased activity in the orientation association area in the parietal lobe. The decreased activity in the orientation association area is responsible for the sensation of losing one's self or expanding its boundaries.

So, where is the self? Is it a figment of mind produced in cooperation with the brain activity? What is the relation between the brain and the body? How does the trio of brain, body and the self-work?

While one may include the Newberg and d'Aquili studies also under the rubric of neural reductionism, in their own claim, they are not exactly dualists or reductionists. While Descartes considers body and mind to be completely separate, Damasio (1994) considers mind as a derivative of brain function, and Newberg and d'Aquili hold the view that while mind is derived from the brain, 'interaction is much more complex and intriguing' (2001, p. 191).

9.2 Neural Correlates Versus Self-correlates

In conjunction with the idea of embodied living that we use today to explain and understand much of human actions, the question that arises is about the locale of the self. Where is the self placed to aid embodiment? Is 'embodied living' the best way to 'understand' consciousness? Is consciousness better understood, as far as its core essence is concerned, by the possibility of non-embodiment? Consciousness functions through the self as self-awareness, self-other-awareness and self-other-awareness' awareness (a third level of awareness that reflects on one's theory of mind). Does the third level warrant a non-embodied state? On the contrary, does metaphysical mysticism that upholds redemption from the body (disembodied states) such as liberation of the self-disregard the significance of embodied living and the sensitivities of the self? These central queries also invite us to conjecture on the order of the placement for the brain, mind, and consciousness, and the relation of each with the self. Is the self located in the brain, or consciousness, or both? Are the locality of the self and non-locality of consciousness mutually tenable?

Another side of the brain-self interaction is the presence of reified human expressions such as empathy, which I would like to term as a 'self-correlate'. Why empathy? Is there an evolutionary advantage for favouring mirror neurons? Empathy and love create extended meanings for the self's existence and experience. The plasticity of the brain teaches the self to make sense, every time, of the change. The brain together with the self perfects the art of transformation and adaptation. The cases of neuropsychiatric patients, subjects with spinal cord injuries and impaired proprioceptive capabilities, who make sense of their oddities, invoke a deeper dimension of the self which is the core and is unnamed. Our ability to self-reflect in deeper ways, and discover new meanings causes wellbeing. Just as we assume that there are neural correlates of consciousness, it might also be reckoned that consciousness has self-correlates. Self-correlates are reified capacities such as empathy, self-reflection and abidance in a core-self. We experience and recognize the smaller versions of self-correlates in the mechanisms of the many neuronal maps that are translated through the complex abilities and sensitivities of the body. Body, in a way, is a smaller reflection of the core-self.

9.3 Beyond the Brain and the Body

If not otherwise asked, the notion of the body is something given and natural to us. But perplexity arises, not just in terms of understanding, but even experiencing, when we reflect upon the possessor, user and witness of the body. The very first thought on these three relations brings to us the question of embodiment. Is embodiment the primary experience bound by certain extremities, such as the exteriority of the skin and the interiority of the private mind? Is embodiment that which gives us the distinction of 'outside-inside' and 'yours-mine', both fine-tuned by a distinct sense of 'me' and 'the rest of the world' (other)? The sense of the body—does it ensue from the basic distinction of 'me and the rest', or is it the other way round—does the distinction of me and the other arise from the sense of the body (however much inclusive or exclusive it is)?

The major limits of current takes on embodiment are: the overt focus on a concept of the body, to retain the conceptual structure of the body without its physicality, and to place the possibility of transcendence as a property of embodied structures and events.

The idea of the body in much of the cognitive science literature is skewed and restricted being mostly limited to functional representationalism and contextual body acts. The Platonic dual worlds theory, Cartesian mind body interaction, the Chalmersian easy problems and hard problem divide, which imply dualism and exclusivity of the *res extensa* and *res cogitans*, continue to influence theories of mind and body.

In the Western world a focused discussion on embodiment started with the post-modernistic age inspired by Humanistic psychology. Humanistic psychology explores the issue of embodiment (Zaner 1971) with emphasis on human perception. Merleau-Ponty stated that the perceiving mind is an 'incarnated mind' (Merleau-Ponty 1964) and Polanyi believed in 'tacit' knowing, and 'knowing other minds and knowing objects' (Polanyi 1966). Later, bringing together the nuances of Buddhist thinking and cognitive sciences, Varela introduced 'embodied action' (Varela et al. 1991).

For an alternate perspective let us discuss the Vedantic notion of *Jiva*, the equivalent of an embodied self, in brief. The Vedantic notion of *Jiva* tries to explain the issue of embodiment in the context of what I wish to call 'enworldment', situated within the larger question of the experienced world. Embodiment is secondary to 'enworldment', since from a macrocosmic view the world is the body (*vapus*) of god. Embodiment is understood in the context of enworldment. For Vedanta, embodiment is the means to realize the never-bodied nature of pure consciousness, which is the core-self. The Vedantic notion of three bodies[1] and embodiments breaks through the either-or aporia. For Vedanta the dualist perspective emerges from the point of view of the body and is not a valid one from the point of view of *Atman* (pure consciousness). The inside-outside view is from the point of view of the body and not pure consciousness. This does not mean that the hierarchy is real, or, in the hierarchy pure consciousness is at the top. The emphasis is on subjectivity that is embodied by a liberated person. Embodied liberation, *jivanmukti*, according to Vedanta is centring the body in pure consciousness, and not the other way. Embodiment is viewed from the point of view of a complex and 'networked body-system'.[2] Vedanta's take on 'embodied

[1] According to Vedanta, there are three bodies of every individual: physical, subtle, and causal bodies.

[2] Swami Bodhananda, a teacher of Vedanta, in conversation with the author in June 2012.

subjectivity' retains the somatic expressions of the body, while invoking a 'pure subjectivity' by going beyond personal identity, which is framed exclusively by life-sustaining bodily functions.

Today, when much of phenomenology-inspired cognitive sciences have saved the 'body' from being just a tissue-muscle physical thing to something more subjective, one is still stuck with the notion of a discrete, disconnected and deconstructed body whose agency is defined around exclusive cognitive and neural functions rather than organismic expressions. A perspective like that of Vedanta, which focuses on transcendence that ensues from pure consciousness (and not embodiment) presents the concept of body afresh.

9.3.1 The Core-Self

The idea of a core-self and its existence have been differently theorized and interpreted by scientists and therapists. I use the core-self to mean the deep organic self that is not influenced by the physical, mental or social self. Core-self is a space of consciousness without forms and names and is the source of healing. Much of the discussions on the body and embodiment have hijacked the possibility and presence of the core-self, which is non-embodied and non-ideated. Core-self is not an emergent or minimal entity that is dependent on the body and bodily functions, but it expresses through them.

Without a concept of the core-self, therapy and healing of disrupted minds is almost impossible. Psychotherapists go beyond the physical, neural, and at times even the mental, to put together the disintegrated mind into one whole, which leads to the person's growth and wellbeing. The major limitation of body-centred theories and approaches such as embodied cognition and embodied action is that something that is physical and hence mortal is given an immortal status. The overt need to preserve the body and bodily concepts is perhaps a response to the traditions and classic theories that have viewed body with apprehension and doubt. But recent attempts have also brought in the metaphysical elevation of the body to a non-corporeal entity, which it is obviously not. The concept of the core-self will help to critique in a healthy fashion the overdone fascination in using the body and embodiment to explain all that is human and humanly actions, and to bring in metaphysical clarity with the highlight on a spiritual non-corporeal presence.

Several cognitive therapists today recognize the importance of experiential learning to ground conceptual learning in the body in order to create new experiential references and habits. Recent studies in neuropsychology also suggest that changing core beliefs is directly related to the experience of the self (Cole 1998, 2004; Ramachandran 1998). The self-narrative of *jivanmukta*, the Vedantic ideal of a self liberated from the world, suggests that the ideal state of liberation is not a disembodied state or an additional acquisition but that which involves a change in the experiential references and the concept of the 'other'. For that reason, embodiment for a *jivanmukta* is situated in the world, in enworldment, and is not necessarily in the giving up or acquisition of the body and its acts thereof. The integral unity conceived for human embodiment is best understood when it is lived and experienced with the focus on the core-self.

9.3.2 Emotion, Its and Our Future

In the last two decades, a visible change that has taken place in the cognitive sciences and neuropsychology is the welcoming of emotions into theorizing and continued inclusion of the unconscious. Affective neuroscience and information system models approach emotions with difference. Linguistic approaches have come to recognize the role of emotions in metaphorical thinking and symbol forming.

From being a sheer processor of information, the mind has taken a new avatar of a complex entity that uses logical structures through its emotions to make effective decisions and define wellbeing. That no experience is meaningful without its extension in time and for which an emotional attribute is necessary is unarguable. Emotion primarily places an experience within a personal context, and subsequently in a social context, without both of which the pleasure of living that is central to human life is impossible.

Though in academic fora we mockingly sideline the valuable inner content of our individual lives by the moniker ‘folk psychology’, the insights that emerge from the stories we tell ourselves about our inner readings are pivotal in construing a valid theory of consciousness. Experiences and their components cannot be understood without the relevance of the person who owns them. It is the *person* who creates and recreates experiences. The enigma of consciousness is the live immediacy that accompanies our experience. Livingston writes: ‘despite the significant methodological shift from the foundationalist epistemology of the 1920s to today’s functionalist explanations of the mind, the problem of explaining consciousness has remained the problem of analysing or describing the logical and relational structure of immediate, given experience’ (Livingston 2002, p. 15).

Historically, the focus on emotions and their immediacy in experiences has been avoided in scientific theorizations. This is due to the general apprehension of such focus causing mental conflicts, and not bearing upon logical reasoning. D.L. Smith remarks:

> Evolutionary theory holds that reproduction is the wellspring and motor of all life, including psychological life. Darwinian explanations of psychological phenomena ultimately involve specifying how a person’s psychological tendencies subserved their reproductive interests in the prehistoric past. The Darwinian emphasis on reproduction sits very well with the centrality of sexual desire in the Freudian system. Furthermore, many of the topics investigated by sociobiologists and evolutionary psychologists, such as self-deception, sexuality and aggression, are also crucial to the Freudian conception of human nature (Smith 2003, p. 57).

The question that is pending and is of significance is, can we have markers of emotions in the self, and for emotions can we shift the focus of biology from the body to the self? In the past decade, Damasio, LeDoux, Panksepp, and others have brought back emotion to the forefront but in the form of the 'unconscious' or pre-reflexive cortical functions, and as something that can be marked in the ancient midbrain and neural circuits.

The divide that James suggested between emotion and feeling is highlighted in recent approaches, and emotion is given a superior place by its contribution to the unconscious processing of information and the emergence of feeling. It is important to consider whether the use of the idea of 'unconscious' by Freud and by the recent neuropsychologists relays the same meaning.

> The term 'unconscious' can cover a multitude of concepts and, as Wittgenstein felicitously put it, if one wraps various pieces of furniture in enough paper, they all end up looking the same (Smith 2003, p. 86).

Recent discussions in affective neuroscience make empirically detailed observations of emotions, and as prevalent in all mammals. Panksepp explains that the presence of emotions in the unconscious is verified by 'primary-process affective states' (in humans and other mammals) which do not require 'neocortical reflective capacities'.

> ... [T]he traditional construct of the dynamic unconscious introduced by Sigmund Freud, is not completely unconscious—it is not totally bereft of experiences. It feels like something to be in primary-process emotional states. We can now be confident that all mammals *experience* their emotions although most, just like newborn human infants, probably do not reflect on these *anoetic* experiences. They may not be cognitively *aware* that they are experiencing feelings; they simply experience such powers as guiding forces of their lives. It is worth emphasizing that although the basic mechanisms of learning may be deeply unconscious, shifting affective feelings (e.g. generating reinforcement effects) on which much of behavioural learning is based are not (Panksepp et al. 2012, p. 13).

Freud used the unconscious in a topographic manner in his attempt to model the mind and to further liberate the agent. Mainstream cognitive science uses the concept of the unconscious to distinguish it from the conscious side of the mental awareness and its contents. For instance, in *Vision,* the well-known book by David Marr (2010), the description of how visual information is unconsciously processed in matter of a second relies not on the conflict and emotion-laden aspect of the unconscious but only on its design and functional role. Smith scathingly points out the difference:

> Cognitive scientists almost always study mental states that are unrelated to emotion and conflict, and which are incapable of becoming conscious because of their very nature, whereas psychoanalysts are usually concerned with conflict laden, emotionally charged unconscious fantasies and memories that are actively excluded from consciousness by the force of repression.... We are not aware of the working of our livers, not because these are repressed or otherwise censored from the slate of consciousness; our unconsciousness of our livers is just an aspect of our design (Smith 2003, pp. 52–53).

In classical psychoanalytic methods, emotion is a key component base whose excess and deficiency lead to various ailments. Emotions are considered to have an impact upon our social relations and self-perceptions. Emotion is foundational in the construction of the self and is a key determinant of self-organization

(Greenberg 2002, p. 87). Such is the relevance of understanding the role of emotions in diagnosing disorders that we have over two centuries of literature on emotion-related symptoms and emotion-related disturbances that characterize disorders.

> Given the ubiquity of emotion-related symptoms in psychopathology (e.g., anger, anhedonia, anxiety, excited mood, fear, flat affect, guilt, irritability, sad mood), most of the early research sought to describe emotion-related disturbances. This work helped to characterize disorders that involve excesses of emotion (e.g., specific phobia, mania), deficits in emotion (e.g., antisocial personality disorder), mismatches between the expression and experience of emotion (e.g., schizophrenia), and deficits in social emotions (e.g., autism)… (Kring 2010, p. 25).

Though emotion is one of the immediate components of our day-to-day experiences, and we believe that distinct emotions are perceived by us through the feelings we receive and give, we have in excess and dearth, neuroscience of emotion has much less to offer on the locale of emotions discretely placed in the brain. The classic perception of the schism between affect and reason,[3] and the view that emotion is controlled by right hemisphere and the logical brain by left brain are not much in vogue. It is increasingly recognized that the processes behind emotion and reason may not be solitary, but interconnected.

An agreed upon perception currently in neuroscience is that like many other functions such as cognition and memory, emotion is also controlled by brain not from a single locus or by a single process, but that both the locus and processes are spread out. Emotion influences many other psychological phenomena and capabilities such as decision-making and consequential thinking. As discussed earlier (in Chap. 7), the concept of 'somatic marker' developed by Damasio has brought to light how emotions reason out our decision-making. We experience emotions in the same manner that we see colour or the way we perceive behaviours in others (Barrett 2006b, p. 20). According to Barrett, we use knowledge to parse and conceptualize the bottom-up information that is sensorially given. The unavoidable connection emotions have to the phenomenal nature of consciousness inspires science to ask new questions on emotion. Some of those questions for a paradigm shift in emotion studies are:

> A new scientific paradigm for the study of emotion means conducting better studies with better research tools. More important, it also means learning to ask different sorts of questions about emotion. In the past, the field has been shaped by questions such as 'Is X an emotion?' 'How many emotions are there?' 'Which specific pattern of antecedent events, neural activity, physiology, and motor behavior defines each emotion?' 'How do we evoke pure instances of emotion, uncontaminated by contextual influences?' and 'How do we regulate and control emotions after they have been triggered?' Conceptual challenges to

[3] Robert Pirsig's famous novel *Zen and the art of motorcycle maintenance* (1975) presents two personalities: one who is mostly interested in the Gestalt and in the moment, and the other to know the details and analysis of the mechanics. Earlier, in the 1950s, Roger Sperry with his student Michael Gazzaniga (Gazzaniga et al. 1962) suggested the lateralization of brain function and that each hemisphere is an independent, conscious system with secluded functions.

> these kinds of questions are met with accusations about denying the biological or evolutionary nature of emotion or even denying the existence of emotion. Emotional responding exists, can be functional, and is very likely given to us by evolution. But that does not necessarily mean that anger, sadness, and fear are useful categories for conducting science.
>
> … An alternative paradigm need not deny the existence of emotions, but might deny emotions any explanatory power. A new paradigm would not deny the importance of evolutionarily preserved responses, but might deny emotions any privileged status as innate neural circuits or modules (Barrett 2006a, p. 47, 49).

Today, there is a change in the conceptualization of emotions exclusively to theorize and diagnose emotion-related disorders. Emotion research has gained unprecedented significance in the context of understanding not just the disorders of mind, but also the brain and organic human capabilities. A shift has occurred from a focus on the relation between psychopathology and emotion, to emotion as a generic mental phenomenon that influences other capabilities. The listing of a basic and limited number of emotions (Ortony and Turner 1990) and emotions as discrete entities and unique patterns of somatovisceral changes (Barrett 2006b) can be questioned. Emotions are seen as less discrete and finished entities but as interactive systems. Both bodily and conceptual components are linked in emotion.

> A given instance of a memory, personality, or concept, is sensitive to context, so may be somewhat different from what occurs at some other instance. This variability, rather than being viewed as a source of error or bias, is a valid reflection of a person's psychological state that must be modeled and explained (Barrett 2006b, p. 21).

With the welcoming of neuroimaging and better conceptualizations, the day will not be far when we can develop a combined somatic, mental, affective and creative approach to emotion. The dimensional and interactive systems model that Barrett et al. suggest might alter the conservative view on emotion as a trait solely impaired in disorders, to start viewing treatment and therapy to bring in 'emotional skills' in addition (Sloan 2006). Contrary to considering emotion as a marker to diagnose mental disorders in psychopathology, in our personal lives, we know that emotions play a key role in contributing to the meaning of our experiences and the balancing of detached, rational assessments.

But then we all do not convey and express our emotions in equal terms. Calling this 'emotional differentiation' and 'emotional granularity', Barrett (2004) says that while some of us use discrete emotional terms, others describe their emotions in generic and global terms.

And though our self-reports might have a distinct description, it is not scientifically possible to qualify different emotions as distinct emotions. We are compelled by own experiences to believe that such and such emotions exist as natural-kind entities. But there is no concrete study yet that gives a strong evidentiary basis for this common belief. There is no clear, unambiguous criterion for indicating the presence of anger or sadness or fear. Addressing this phenomenon as 'emotion paradox', Barrett writes: 'The taxonomic structure of self-reported experiences of emotion does not support the view that anger, sadness, fear, and so on, are qualitatively distinct and experientially primitive' (Barrett 2006b, p. 25).

Owing to the scenario that our self-reports about emotions for ourselves or others contain insufficient or inaccurate representation, or, the emotions we report can themselves be another, and that till date there has been no pinpointed neuroscientific correlate of emotion mapped in the brain or body for each distinct emotion, it is prudent to suppose that the distinctness of emotions as we perceive them is alterable. One of the best examples of such a possibility is from emotion-focused therapy, where the role of emotion coaches (therapists) is to help the client become aware of, accept and make sense of their emotional experience (Greenberg 2002). The fundamental principle of emotion therapy involves the transformation of one emotion into another (Greenberg 2006). For instance, a maladaptive emotional state can be transformed by undoing it with an adaptive emotion, or a negative emotion can be undone by a positive emotion (Frederickson 2001).

Darwin (1872), LeDoux (1998), Panksepp (2005) and others have sided on a theory of emotion that favours biological and social functions. They also ask if basic emotions such as anger, sadness, fear, etc., are caused by distinctive neural circuitries. Barrett (2006b, p. 43) argues that since neuroimaging studies in humans are only just now beginning to develop methods to map the neural circuitry within the human brain, this question remains unanswered.

The propounder of a body-centric envisioning of emotions, William James, said with no ambiguity that emotion is the unconscious biological process in the body, but feeling is experienced. But whether James' focus on bodily associations of emotions has to be understood differently is another debatable issue. Barrett argues that although James' writings are laced with detailed descriptions of the bodily symptoms that characterize anger, grief, fear, and the like, he explicitly stated in several places that variability within each emotion category is the norm and that he rejected the idea that a single set of bodily symptoms could describe all instances of a given emotion category across individuals (Barrett 2006b, p. 42).

Damasio (1999, 2003), Ledoux (1998) suggested that emotions are the covert somatic processes that happen inside the body even before we feel them. And every emotion is marked in the body and influences future actions of the person. Many social psychologists also consider the covert nature of emotion to be more convincing. For instance, Franks (2007) remarks that emotion is the ineffable language of the body in contrast to the linguistic language of the mind and counts two reasons that the emotional unconscious is important for social psychology.

> … [T]he neuronal channels going up from the emotional centers of the brain to the more cognitive centers are denser and more robust than the cognitive centers going down to inhibit and control the emotional structures. Self-conscious efforts to avoid prejudice, fear, hatred, and depression are often rendered unsuccessful by this imbalance. Second is the consistent finding that unconscious preferences and emotional leanings exert significantly more influence over our thoughts and behaviors than do conscious preferences (Franks 2007, p. 39).

The leaning of social psychology and mainstream neuroscience towards the unconscious portrayal of human emotions—though it might be conducive to build upon the evolutionary and social function theories—greatly dismisses the quality of human consciousness that can rise against bodily engravings, and express freedom and conscious alterations. That the unconscious processing of emotion itself takes cues from conscious experiences and feelings also suggests that it is time that we moved ahead from distinguishing between emotion and feeling to favour the coexistence of biological processes and the affective content of emotions. For instance, Barrett says:

> Although there are a number of methodological and theoretical factors that currently limit our ability to draw inferences about the neural bases of emotional responses, the failure to find neural signatures for distinct emotions thus far is consistent with the behavioral evidence (Barrett 2006b, p. 23).
>
> … emotions may not be real categories with mechanisms that are hardwired into the brain, waiting to be found with better research tools (Barrett 2006a, b, p. 42).
>
> If emotions are psychological events like memories, then they are best thought of as products of distinct but interacting psychological processes with accompanying neural systems, and scientists might begin to design experiments to systematically map how instances of emotion are synthesized from component psychological processes that we know to be implemented in the human brain. Doing so may provide us with a better translation of the pages of 'nature's infinite book' that are the workings of the brain, and allow us to answer the age-old question of what emotions really are (Barrett and Wager 2006, p. 83).

Though the somatic processes are not presented to us, we are certainly aware of and are influenced by our feelings. To divide affect into emotion and feeling, unconscious and conscious events, will also pose questions about the nature of desires we form, attitudes we have, and identities we develop. Further, feelings cannot be reduced to an emergent phenomenon of processing that happens in an unconscious level, since all that which we are informed of at a point is through conscious feelings. We know our bodies through feelings. Feelings help us weigh our judgements. Our knowledge about our selves is traversed by our feelings. Hence, as Madell and Ridley (1997, p. 149) quip, feeling cannot be regarded as a pure epiphenomenon, a sort of affective varnish which could be cleaned off without serious consequences. Madell critiques also the view about feelings as a set of judgements. It is the 'notion of *feeling towards* which is fundamental to an acceptable account of emotion, and of value' (Madel, p. 160). The stark point of view that he propounds is that emotion cannot be in the realm of the unconscious. The phenomenological and the affective are salient to consciousness. Emotions, desire and pleasure are states that are indissolubly both intentional and affective.

Cognitive engagement with the world is possible through our affective orientation (Madell and Ridely 1997, p. 174). Shanahan (2008) proposes an integrated model of emotions and motivations, furthering the ideas of Karl Pribram, to show how emotions may have contributed to the emergence of symbolic formation and ultimately to every aspect of language. The renewed approach to emotions and their place in the study of brain brings forth the other side of the human that is distanced from cognition and the unconscious, though both continue to influence our views, even by being annoyingly persistent.

9.3.3 Enactment and Therapy

The role of emotion in therapy is centuries old. And the use of emotion in producing an aesthetic and artistic favour, too, is as ancient as the beginning of human times. One of the recent methods in therapy that uses art is 'drama therapy'. Drama therapy[4] believes in the extraordinary relation between the therapist and the client that results in bringing about the client's healing. This method is also wary of the dangers involved in the limits of such a relationship and the possibility of the Freudian transference usurping the intended goal. An experiment in drama therapy called 'developmental transformations' uses the play space, encounter, and embodiment to bring out healing. It uses embodied encounter with another person to bring about the contact with the core-self.

> In Developmental Transformations, the core-Self is distinguished from personality and is considered of equal importance to it. Developmental Transformations therapists believe that personal identity is constructed by a series of roles and narratives that defines one's persona but that underneath these masks or structures is a core-Self that is related to a sense of Being....Developmental Transformations theory extends beyond an ego-based psychology to include aspects of transpersonal psychology.... Access or contact with this core-Self occurs through the body and energy (Porter 2000, p. 311).

The tradition of yoga is known to use the body and embodiment to establish oneself in a non-embodied space of consciousness. Drama therapy to a great extent embraces metaphysical dualism and places both core-self and body as indispensable and mutually irreducible to each other. Following the co-dependence of the self and the body, and one's own body and another's, it believes healing to be relational and something that requires a 'relationship to exist between the therapist and client in order for growth to occur in treatment' (Porter 2000).

One of the central beliefs of drama therapy draws from the natural urge of humans since time immemorial to represent another object or person through drawings, play acts, rituals, dance, sculpture, etc. Both in enactment and therapy there is an attempt to draw from the inner space of the person, to bring it to the forefront, and use it for personal and collective wellbeing. Since the goal is to address a wholesome individual, experiential therapies that use forms of art would like to call the method not a 'technique' but a 'process' (Robbins et al. 1979). The 'process'-oriented approach to therapy and life facilitates a much required trait:

---

[4] Drama therapy is defined by the National Association for Drama Therapy as '... the systematic and intentional use of drama/theatre processes, products, and associations to achieve the therapeutic goals of symptom relief, emotional and physical integration and personal growth.' Drama therapy is an active approach that helps the client tell their story to solve a problem, achieve a catharsis, extend the depth and breadth of inner experience, understand the meaning of images, and strengthen the ability to observe personal roles while increasing flexibility between roles. Drama therapy evolved from the experience and research of psychotherapists, teachers and theater professionals who recognized that alternatives to traditional verbal therapies were useful to permit clients to confront, explore and work through problems and emotional difficulties.' See http://www.dramatherapyinstitutela.com/creativemainframe.htm.

openness that would question the rigidity of refined, close-ended, reductive, and minimalistic approaches to human consciousness.

Take, for instance, the oldest text in the world on theatre and aesthetics, from India, called *Natyasastra*. There is elaborate discussion, on one hand, on the characteristics of playhouse, plays, complex gestures and movements, rules of prosody, metres and music, use of languages, style of characters, costumes and ornaments. And, on the other, there is elaboration on emotions and mental states, mutuality of emotions and mental states, rapport between actor and spectator, mental and physical characteristics of the actor and spectator, preliminary mystic rituals for effective representation and final goals of drama. In the text, there is a structural rigidity as to the epistemology, and openness about subjectivity, and relationship between the actor and the spectator.

The text addresses three levels of open-ended complexity: joint participation of gesture and movements, mental states and emotions; relationship between the actor and the spectator, of the actor invoking a specific state of emotion in the spectator's mind; and the spontaneous and self-evolving nature of enjoyment for the audience (Menon 2003). The rigorous and specified rules of *natya* (performance), together with the first-person experience of the actor and the spectator, in *Natyasastra* provide a wholesome representation of human emotions through the complex act of the physical body (gestures, costumes, music and plot) and the spiritual body (emotions, states of mind, and unique relationship between the one who is presenting the representation and one who is enjoying it). *Natyasastra* and drama therapy relocate the body from the physical to the non-physical framework, and invoke the non-corporeal nature of the core-self.

The shift of the focus from the body and its embodied adherents to the core-self has to take recourse to the method of both the body and the core-self. The liberation of the body, its extensions, and the acceptance of its limits has to happen with a simultaneous reckoning of the core-self and its essential non-dependence on the body.

9.4 Self in the Brain and Brain in the Self

Given the overwhelming rule of the brain over the human body and mind, can the way we act, think and make decisions be altered by understanding the human brain? Brain studies in participation with a score of disciplines, including religious and spiritual teachings, anticipate the possibility of changes in the experience of the self. Studies on neural dysfunctions, affective neuroscience, art-mind relations, and spiritual experiences reveal not only the possibility of major cognitive and motor changes, but also changes in self-perception and self-expression. The regenerative nature of the brain throws open exciting challenges for all engaged in knowing the human self better.

It is the brain's evolutionary development that has paved way for our thinking capabilities in terms of abstract symbols like language, and building up knowledge through generations. There are three important aspects to the nature of brain function. These are: (1) various cortical areas are demarcated for highly specialized functions, providing a brain map for the locations of functions; (2) different brain areas work in unison and harmony; and (3) though the sensory and motor functions are localized, the brain possesses the ability to transfer, extend, and take over functions (as in the case of new learning; eventualities of neural deafferentation due to stroke; artistic capabilities; mystic and spiritual experiences). The regenerative nature of the brain has made it the 'smart organ', which seems to have an inherent intelligence with its flexible nature.

The brain is a flexible organ, described by neurologists as 'plasticity'. This most significant characteristic of the brain makes it possible to rewire and redefine concepts. As we learn we change the structure of the brain. Each time we learn a word a reconnection is made between the nerve cells. As we acquire knowledge a rewiring is made in the brain. The self-healing and open nature of the brain enables it to transfer functions to different areas when a specific cortical area dysfunctions due to stroke. The left side of the brain of a right-handed person specializes in enabling music, poetry and mathematics. After hemispherectomy, these capabilities travel from the left to the right side of the brain; though it is now known that the ability to transfer functions is highest before adolescence.

Contrary to traditional, deterministic theory, current extensive research performed by scientists worldwide proves that the brain develops, learns and grows depending upon the interaction between the person and environment, and in response to challenges. Brain research is increasingly documenting cases where the brain promotes activity in one region to overcome the loss in another region. The brain is capable of forming new neural networks and favour new learning.

Further, it is now understood that the development of the brain is not linear. The theory that the capacity of the brain to learn increases as an infant matures into adulthood and thereafter declines is challenged by current research findings. The non-linear nature of the brain's development is being discussed with enthusiasm. Acquisition of knowledge and skills do not happen in a linear fashion but at optimal times. The brain continues to grow and form new neural networks until death if there are optimal environmental conditions and appropriate training (Schwartz and Begley 2002). Alongside, there is another finding that the brain degenerates if it is not used. If other cells do not appropriately stimulate a cell, it self-destructs. This self-destruction process is also known to be an important factor in strokes, Alzheimer's and motor neuron diseases, leading to the loss of essential nerve cells from the adult brain.

The structural anatomy of the brain, and the course of its functioning, highlights exciting issues for debate and reflection. These are centred on the subjective and self-preserving nature of the brain. It is baffling to think that the brain is capable of not just change and growth but can also change its course as a self-preserving system, and 'reflect' upon that course with the help of cues from the self, which is located nowhere, or perhaps everywhere. It facilitates the mind to think, imagine and direct action according to newer and challenging contexts.

Perhaps it might be a quick jump to assume that such a nature of the brain indicates a mind that is owned by a self. The hard problem of consciousness persisted through the 'decade of the brain' and is closing in for another decade. Yet, the problem has only vetted newer and newer responses without offering a resolution. Why and how the quantitative structural inputs of the brain give rise to physical outputs, which are possessed and housed by a self, whose contours are frilled by deeply subjective qualities, remain a riddle for twenty-first century science. The self is capable of being hurt not just physically (through the body), but also mentally. The physical pain is even controlled, transcending the overpowering neural influence, by the mental and spiritual qualities that are developed or possessed naturally.

Damasio's efforts to prove Descartes' dualism wrong, and Todd Feinberg's proposal for 'compositional or nested hierarchy' (Feinberg 2001, p. 127), suggests that the self and the subjective nature of experience are not issues to be dispensed through simple naturalistic theories. Perhaps we need to study better the finer aspects of higher human faculties such as introspection, reflection and contemplation. In mainstream neuroscience, generally the discussion is focused on a fractured self, a self impaired by neurological dysfunctions, or a segregated self. The self discussed from such a perspective is already limited to a certain disposition. Self-ascriptions are about the self that is impaired, or valid only in a discrete context. Such an approach takes away the wholesome personality out of context, and focuses on the dissociative or hallucinating self. There is no adequate discussion on subsequent experiences once the impairment is intervened or cured. Perhaps anticipating this significant issue, Metzinger says:

> The issue is not only how a phenomenal self per se can arise but how beings like us come to use this phenomenal self as a tool for experiencing themselves as subjects. We need interdisciplinary answers to questions like these: What does it mean that in conscious experience we are not only *related to the world*, but related to it *as knowing selves*? What, exactly, does it mean that a phenomenal self typically is not only present in an experiential reality but that at the same time it forms the *center* of this reality? How do we come to think and speak about ourselves as *first persons*? (Metzinger 2003, p. 6).

To limit the self-brain interactions to linear and physical processes would foreclose the richness and possibilities that lie hidden. The self-challenged brain and the brain-challenged self-reinforce, change, and adjust each other. And through these 'adjustments' they create meaning and purpose that we constantly experience in our lives. We might say that the self is the possibility for the brain to look 'inward', and the brain is the vantage point for the self to look 'outward'—a mutually balancing process. Perhaps, it is through their complex interrelations that we understand both.

The pursuit of human knowledge has been guided by the practise of locating it in a space and time. This trend has definitely proven successful in brain science to a greater extent. The major baffle that brain scientists face is the curious play that the brain engages with the self—its tremendous capacity to change its structure by way of creating more neurons, storing new learning in memory, and changing the neural networks moving away from trodden neural spaces. There is no one genetically aligned way the brain follows. There is something which 'tells' the brain to change if optimal conditions are available. The brain seems to be a continuously adapting 'agent'. Or can the brain be the agent all by itself? Can the agenthood be attributed to a physical system?

The multiple intelligence theory of Howard Gardner (1983) says that every individual has one or more of seven distinct types of intelligences, such as linguistic, logical-mathematical, bodily kinaesthetic, spatial, musical, interpersonal and intrapersonal. According to Gardner, to ask where intelligence is located is like asking 'Where is the voice situated in the radio?'. Intelligence is a capacity. In a similar sense, could the self be a capacity in collaboration with the brain, not located anywhere? But then the nature of self is prone to the disposition of its beholder and is hence differently unique. Even if we concede with this hypothesis, the problem of subjectivity looms large. There seems to be a core-self that is marked by hope, love and human sensitivities. These are not just psychological qualities. They are able to defy physical conditions and present independently without a physical basis.

Consciousness studies has heralded all along that the brain is the basis for consciousness, and consciousness can be traced to different areas of the brain. While definitely the role of brain, and also the functional specificities embedded in different neuronal patches cannot be undermined, the idea that the brain is the cause of consciousness is unacceptable to those who believe in the greater power of the human self. A recent paper published in *Journal of Consciousness Studies* (Majorek 2012) provides a scathing criticism against neural reductionism with the help of gaps in empirical studies and conceptual assumptions behind the idea that the brain causes conscious experience. Marek Majorek argues:

> A pianist cannot play a piano concerto when his piano gets damaged, or at least his performance is impaired by the damage to his instrument. Yet it would be absurd to claim that the piano is the cause of the concerto. It is merely *a necessary condition* for its performance, not its cause. Similarly, it is a fallacy to claim that the loss of a mental function as a result of brain damage *proves* that the brain plays the causal role in producing this mental function. It is a fallacy to take a merely (under normal circumstances) *necessary* condition of an event to be the *cause* of this event, for a cause of an event is not identical with a necessary condition of it. It may very well be that the brain is (under normal circumstances) a necessary condition for consciousness, but this does not prove that it is its cause. The brain may turn out to be a mere piano on which some pianist is able to play her concert (Majorek 2012, p. 129).

We begin with the theory that the brain creates the self. But then at some point the self starts influencing the brain. There is a reverse influence violating the classical causal route. The *self-in-the-brain* and *brain-in-the-self* influence each other to create adaptability for new scenarios. With self-effort brain creates new neural networks. With new learning one receives hope that further encourages brain functions. Can we presume that it is the core-self which makes the effort, whose brain is influenced by hope, who tells the brain to change and adapt?

Do we experience, or have access to a core-self, which is not related to the self that is assembled by and filtered through the brain?

Can I have a self in spite of my brain and my embodiment? It is not at all easy to answer this question either in the affirmative or negative.

In our analysis of which part of the self remains after brain death, we make a sort of category mistake. The concept of the self that is understood in a scientific discussion is a composite of neural, emotional and behavioural aspects. When death occurs there is no way to understand these aspects in a distinct fashion. While we assume the post-mortem existence of the self in some form, what we forget is that the concept of the self itself has changed with the death of the body. It is no longer the self that we conceived of while the body was alive and which the body expressed it in many ways. Therefore, is it logically correct to assume that a part of the self is left after death though its neural and emotional parts remain absent? If a major chunk of the self is lost (with death), then can we assume some parts of it to remain? These are questions that emerge if our idea of the self is a composite self that is conceived on the basis of life and its expressions.

Should we, the civilized Homo sapiens, also believe, like the ancient Neanderthal, that the self (soul) rises above like the smoke from the fire and goes to the unseen space of the sky? Perhaps not! But the question that is essential for us to ask is: Is there a core-self somehow hidden and which master-controls the living self through the body and the brain? Is that pure consciousness? Is the existence of pure consciousness unhindered by the birth and death of the body?

A short response is that the core-self is beyond the binary of birth and death of the body, and it is the central key to resolve the puzzle of consciousness.

References

Barrett, L. F. (2004). Feelings or words? Understanding the content in self-report ratings of experienced emotion. *Journal of Personality and Social Psychology, 87*, 266–281.

Barrett, L. F. (2006a). Are emotions natural kinds? *Perspectives on Psychological Science, 1*(1), 28–58.

Barrett, L. F. (2006b). Solving the emotion paradox: Categorization and the experience of emotion. *Personality and Social Psychology Review, 10*(1), 20–46.

Barrett, L. F., & Wager, T. D. (2006). The structure of emotion: Evidence from neuroimaging studies. *Current Directions in Psychological Science, 15*(3), 79–83.

Beauregard, V., & Paquette, M. (2006). Neural correlates of a mystical experience in Carmelite nuns. *Neuroscience Letters, 405*(3), 186–190.

Cole, J. (1998). *About Face*. Cambridge, MA: The MIT Press.

Cole, J. (2004). *Still lives: Narratives of spinal cord injury*. London: MIT Press.

Damasio, A. (1994). *Descartes' error: Emotion, reason and the human brain*. New York: G.P. Putnam's Sons.

Damasio, A. (1999). *Feeling of what happens: Body and emotion in the making of consciousness*. London: Heinemann.

Damasio, A. (2003). *Looking for Spinoza: Joy, sorrow and the feeling brain*. London: William Heinemann.

d'Aquili, E., & Newberg, A. (1993). Liminality, trance and unitary states in ritual and meditation. *Studia Liturgica, 23*, 2–34.

Darwin, C. (1872). *The expression of emotions in man and animals*.

Feinberg, T. E. (2001). *Altered egos: How the brain creates the self*. Oxford: Oxford University Press.

Franks, D. D. (2007). The neuroscience of emotions. In J. E. Stets, & J. H. Turner (Eds.), *Handbook of the sociology of emotions* (pp. 38–62). New York: Springer Science.

Frederickson, B. (2001). The role of positive emotions in positive psychology: The broaden-and-build theory of positive emotions. *American Psychologist, 56*(3), 218–226.

Gardner, H. (1983). *Frames of mind.* New York: Basic Book Inc.

Gazzaniga, M. S., Bogen, J. E., & Sperry, R. W. (1962). Some functional effects of sectioning the cerebral commissures in man. *Proceeding of the National Academy of Sciences, 48* (Part 2), 1765–1769.

Greenberg, L. (2002). *Emotion-focused therapy: Coaching clients to work through feelings.*

Greenberg, L. (2006). Emotion-focused Therapy: A synopsis. *Journal of Contemporary Psychotherapy, 36,* 87–93.

Kelly, E. F., Kelly, E. W., Crabtree, A., Gauld, A., Grosso, M., & Greyson, B. (2007). *Irreducible mind: Toward a psychology for the 21st century.* Plymouth: Rowman and Littlefield Publishers. Inc.

Kozart, M. (1998). Religious experience was not correctly defined. *Journal of Neuropsychiatry and Clinical Neurosciences, 10,* 475.

Kring, A. M. (2010). The future of emotion research in the study of psychopathology. *Emotion Review, 2*(3), 225–228.

LeDoux, J. (1998). *The emotional brain: The mysterious underpinnings of emotional life.* New York: Simon & Schuster.

Liviingston, P. (2002). Experience and structure: Philosophical history and the problem of consciousness. *Journal of Consciousness Studies, 9*(3), 15–33.

Madell, G., & Ridley, A. (1997). Emotion and feeling. *Proceedings of the Aristotelian Society, 71,* 147–176.

Majorek, M. B. (2012). Does the brain cause conscious experience? *Journal of Consciousness Studies, 19*(3–4), 121–144.

Marr, D. (2010). *Vision: A computational investigation into the human representation and processing of visual information.* New York: The MIT Press.

Menon, S. (2003). Binding experiences for a first person approach: Looking at Indian ways of thinking (darsana) and acting (natya) in the context of current discussions on 'consciousness'. In C. Chakraborti., M. K. Mandal & R. B. Chatterjee (Eds.), *On mind and consciousness* (pp. 90–117). Indian Institute of Advanced Study, Shimla and Department of Humanities and Social Sciences IIT Kharagpur.

Merleau-Ponty, M. (1964). *The primacy of perception.* Evanston: Northwestern University Press.

Metzinger, T. (2003). *Being no one: The self-model theory of subjectivity.* New York: MIT Press.

Newberg, A., d'Aquili, E., & Rause, V. (2001). *Why god won't go away: Brain science and the biology of belief.* New York: Ballantine Books.

Newberg, A., Pourdehnad, M., Alavi, A., & d'Aquili, E. (2003). Cerebral blood flow during meditative prayer: preliminary findings and methodological issues. *Perceptual and Motor Skills,* 97, 625–630.

Ortony, A., & Turner, T. (1990). What's basic about basic emotions? *Psychological Review, 97*(3), 315–331.

Panksepp, J. (2005). On the embodied neural nature of core emotional affects. In G. Colombetti & E. Thompson (Eds.). *Journal of Consciousness Studies, 12*(8–10), 158–184.

Panksepp, J., Asma, S., Curran, G., Gabriel, R., & Greif, T. (2012). The philosophical implications of affective neuroscience. *Journal of Consciousness Studies, 19*(3–4), 6–48.

Polanyi, M. (1966). *The tacit dimension.* London: The University of Chicago Press.

Porter, L. (2000). The bifurcated gift: Love and intimacy in drama psychotherapy. *The Arts in Psychotherapy, 7*(5), 309–320.

Ramachandran, V. A. (1998). *Phantoms in the brain.* New York: William Morrow.

Restak, R. M. (1982). The archaeology of the self. *The Wilson Quarterly, 6*(3), 98–104.

Robbins, A., Adler, S., Eigen, M., Roland, A., Strahl, L., & Wallace, E. (1979). Dialogue in creative and therapeutic growth. *Art Psychotherapy, 6,* 221–232.

Saver, J. L., & Rabin, J. (1997). The neural substrates of religious experiences. *Journal of Neuropsychiatry and Clinical Neurosciences, 9*(3), 498–510.

Schwartz, J. M., & Begley, S. (2002). *The mind and the brain: Neuroplasticity and the power of the mental force*. New York: HarperCollins Publishers.
Shanahan, D. (2008). A new view of language, emotion and the brain. *Integrative Psychological and Behavioural Science, 42*, 6–19.
Sloan, D. M. (2006). The importance of emotion in psychotherapy approaches. *Journal of Contemporary Psychotherapy, 36*, 59–60.
Smith, D. L. (2003). *Psychoanalysis in focus*. In W. Dryden (Ed.). London: Sage Publications.
Varela, F., Thompson, E., & Rosch, E. (1991). *The embodied mind: Cognitive science and human experience*. Cambridge, MA: MIT Press.
Zaner, R. M. (1971). *The problem of embodiment: Some contributions to a phenomenology of the body (phaenomenologica)*. New York: Springer.

Index

S. Menon, *Brain, Self and Consciousness*, Studies in Neuroscience, Consciousness and Spirituality, DOI: 10.1007/978-81-322-1581-3,

W

Z

MIX
Papier aus verantwortungsvollen Quellen
Paper from responsible sources
FSC® C105338

If you have any concerns about our products,
you can contact us on
ProductSafety@springernature.com

In case Publisher is established outside the EU,
the EU authorized representative is:
Springer Nature Customer Service Center GmbH
Europaplatz 3, 69115 Heidelberg, Germany

Printed by Libri Plureos GmbH
in Hamburg, Germany